100 DAYS TO A
YOUNGER
BRAIN

Maximize Your Memory, Boost Your
Brain Health, and Defy Dementia

SABINA BRENNAN

LIFE
LONG

To David, for everything.

_____

Copyright © 2020 by Sabina Brennan
Cover design by Terri Sirma
Cover copyright © 2020 Hachette Book Group, Inc.

Hachette Books
Hachette Book Group
1290 Avenue of the Americas, New York, NY 10104
www.HachetteBooks.com
Twitter.com/HachetteBooks
Instagram.com/HachetteBooks

Printed in the United States of America

First Edition: January 2020

Published by Hachette Books, an imprint of Perseus Books, LLC, a subsidiary of Hachette Book Group, Inc. The Hachette Books name and logo is a trademark of the Hachette Book Group.

The Hachette Speakers Bureau provides a wide range of authors for speaking events. To find out more, go to www.hachettespeakersbureau.com or call (866) 376-6591.

The publisher is not responsible for websites (or their content) that are not owned by the publisher.

Library of Congress Control Number: 2019953839

ISBNs: 978-0-306-84648-9 (trade paperback); 978-0-306-84647-2 (ebook)

LSC-C

10 9 8 7 6 5 4 3 2 1

Contents

Introduction

100 Days to a Younger Brain delivers, in clear everyday language, the basics on how your brain works and how you can keep it healthy, and shares the good news that you can boost brain health and change your brain at any age. As you work through this life-changing program, you will complete a series of assessments to show you a clear picture of the current state of your brain health and give you insight into what you are doing right and what needs fixing.

Whether you've come to this book because you are concerned about your memory, you fear getting dementia, or simply value your brain and want to look after it, you will find an abundance of practical tips within these pages that can easily be incorporated into your daily life. These down-to-earth suggestions will help to rejuvenate your brain, optimize memory performance, boost brain health, and even build resilience to allow your brain to cope with or compensate for aging, injury, and diseases that affect the brain, including dementia.

Your brain is fundamental to who you are and it supports you in the things you do each and every day. Brain health is not a passing fad and, once you think about it, it's quite astonishing that up to now we have essentially excluded our most complex, and most important, organ from our health-care routines.

This is not a book about being brainy but it is a book about being smart enough to invest in brain health. We talk about physical health and we talk about mental health. We even talk about dental health and heart health. It just seemed crazy to me that no one was talking about brain health. After all, you need your brain for *everything*. There isn't one thing that you can do without your brain. Just as you invest time every day in dental health, I hope that this book inspires you to do at least one thing every day to boost your brain health.

I didn't go to university until I was forty-two. Six years later I emerged with a degree in psychology, a PhD, and a passion for brain health. As a cognitive neuroscientist[1] and a director of a dementia research program in the Institute of Neuroscience at Trinity College Dublin, I was involved in, surrounded by, and exposed to incredible brain research. Thanks in no small part to amazing advances in brain-imaging technology, scientists are making phenomenal progress in terms of our understanding of brain function and diseases that affect the brain.

But something troubled me. Scientists were doing great work but they spent much of their time talking to other scientists about their research at niche conferences and in academic journals, most of which are inaccessible to the general public. Of course, this kind of academic discourse is absolutely essential for scientific progress, but the scientific literature and research on brain health and dementia can be complex and not easy for everyone to follow. That's why I've written this book. It translates scientific jargon into easy-to-understand, practical information to improve your brain health.

100 Days to a Younger Brain will show you how to hold on to important functions like memory into old age. Adopting a brain-healthy lifestyle is like investing in brain capital; by making smart choices you can build reserves that you can cash in at some point in the future when faced with a challenge such as aging, injury, or disease.

Let's take Alzheimer's disease.[2] There is currently no cure. The Alzheimer brain is shriveled and atrophied[3] compared to a healthy brain and is characterized by cell death and tissue loss. Nobody knows for sure what causes this cell death, but abnormal protein clusters called plaques and twisted strands of another protein called tangles are currently the prime suspects.

You'd be forgiven for thinking that having these plaques and tangles in your brain would mean that you would have the symptoms that we commonly associate with dementia—such as memory loss and confusion. But you would be wrong. You *can* have the disease in your brain and *not* experience symptoms! And that more than anything inspired me to write this book.

Let me explain. **We know from research that the brains of up to 25 percent of people who have sufficient pathology for a diagnosis of Alzheimer's disease post mortem are clinically intact before death.** About one in four people with the pathology in their brain are resilient to the disease. This means that even though they had the disease, the plaques and tangles, they had no perceptible symptoms. In fact, they remained coherent and continued to function as normal up until they died.

We call this resilience "reserve." Your brain has the capacity for resilience, too, provided you give it a helping hand by adopting a brain-healthy lifestyle. What's more, you can replenish these reserves across your lifespan.

Consider for a moment Jake and Peter, two fifty-five-year-old men. Jake has high reserve (high resilience) and Peter has low reserve (low resilience). Both begin to develop the pathology of Alzheimer's disease in their brains at the same time. For illustrative purposes, let's say that both die at the age of seventy-five.

Peter, the individual with low reserve, will show symptoms of dementia that gradually worsen over the years. The impairment to Peter's cognitive functioning[4] progresses along a gradually declining slope, going from mild through moderate, to severe and ultimately to his death at the age of seventy-five.

In contrast, Jake, the individual with high reserve, won't manifest any perceptible symptoms. The disease pathology is still progressing in Jake's brain but his high levels of reserve allow him to cope with and compensate for the physical damage that is occurring in his brain. Let's say Jake has a fatal accident at seventy-five. When his brain is examined post-mortem he becomes one of the 25 percent who have sufficient pathology in their brain for a diagnosis of dementia but who were clinically cognitively intact at time of death.

Now it is only fair to point out that had Jake not had the misfortune to be run over by an ice-cream van on the way home from his seventy-fifth birthday celebrations his reserves would eventually have been exhausted and he would at some point have manifested dementia symptoms. However, unlike Peter, who had experienced very gradual loss, Jake's decline would be dramatic and severe. Like falling off a cliff edge. At some point in the future—had he lived—Jake would have experienced a precipitous drop in his cognitive functioning, bypassing the mild and moderate stages.

Reserve is not a "golden ticket," nor is it a "get-out-of-jail-free card" but if you build it up through brain-healthy choices, you can defer the onset of dementia symptoms and grant yourself more independent years in possession of your mental faculties.

This resilience isn't just limited to dementia, it can optimize your everyday brain performance and protect your cognitive functions against injury, stroke, and even diseases like multiple sclerosis[5] that strike in early adulthood. Your brain also has an amazing ability to adapt and change across your lifespan. This flexibility, which is called neuro-plasticity,[6] allows you to learn new things, adapt to changes in your life and environment, and also allows you to compensate for disease and injury.

A stroke or "brain attack" occurs when blood flow to an area of the brain is cut off. Spontaneous plastic changes occur in the brain following a stroke that can help the brain to compensate and can contribute significantly to recovery, for example, of movement. The brain compensates for the damage by activating alternative pathways that run parallel to the damaged one. Recovery from stroke involves relearning motor function using the newly activated compensatory pathways. Stroke is the leading cause of acquired disability, and nine out of ten strokes could be prevented by minimizing risk through brain-healthy life choices. There is considerable variability in the extent to which patients recover after stroke. While the reason behind the varied outcomes is not fully clear, lifestyle factors are thought to play a role and you will read more about that in Chapter 1.

This program will also help you to develop brain-healthy habits that could greatly improve outcomes after stroke or brain injury. If you already have a dementia diagnosis or were to develop a disease that affects brain function, such as Alzheimer's or multiple sclerosis, at some point in your future, following this guide and building a bespoke Brain Health Plan will enable you to minimize your symptoms and support your independence while living with the disease. Brain health matters, especially if you consider that one in three older adults will have a stroke, dementia, or both.

I have a mission in life, and that mission is to vastly increase the number of people who are able to build up their resilience to brain diseases, so they can live happier, more independent lives for very much longer. Like any good book I think that the final chapter of life should be one of the best. I want to get you talking and thinking about brain health. I want you to look after your brain as routinely as you look after your teeth.

100 Days to a Younger Brain will change the way you live, guiding you toward brain-healthy choices, arming you with practical advice that you can implement each day to rejuvenate and optimize your brain performance, build up your reserves, increase plasticity, and reduce dementia risk. Now it's time to enjoy the *good news* about brain health.

How To Use This Book

Chapter 1 explains why everyone needs to invest in brain health.

Chapter 2 explains how your brain works and how you can bank reserves to boost brain health.

Chapters 3–8 introduce the program for *100 Days to a Younger Brain*, covering the lifestyle factors that are important for brain health: sleep, stress, social and mental activity, heart health, physical activity, and attitude. As you work through each chapter you will complete a series of assessments that will help you to determine your current brain health profile for each of these factors. The information and assessments in each chapter will help you to set goals and devise an action plan to improve your assets and reduce your risks for each of these lifestyle factors. Where a term has a superscript number (e.g., neuroscientist[1]) you will find further explanation of that term beside the corresponding number in the Notes on page 288.

Chapter 3— **Days 1–7:** *Create your sleep profile and plan*

Chapter 4— **Days 8–14:** *Create your stress profile and plan*

Chapter 5— **Days 15 and 16:** *Create your mental and social profile and plan*

Chapter 6— **Days 17–23:** *Create your heart-health profile and plan*

Chapter 7— **Days 24–30:** *Create your physical activity profile and plan*

Chapter 8— **Days 31 and 32:** *Create your attitude profile and plan*

Chapter 9— **Day 33:** *Create your overall Brain Health Profile*

Day 34: *Build your bespoke Brain Health Plan*

Days 35–100: *Embed the brain-health habit into your daily life and put your plan into action*

Research suggests that it takes on average sixty-six days to introduce a new daily habit, which is why I have allowed that length of time to embed the brain-health habit into your daily routine.

100-Day Diary

Building a daily brain-health habit is critical for success. To help you to do this I have included a 100-Day Diary at the end of the last chapter that you can use to record your brain-healthy actions each day as you work through the program.

You will increase your chances of success if you commit to doing at least one thing each day that is good for your brain health. Set a daily reminder on your phone, on your calendar, or place a Post-it note on your fridge or beside your toothbrush to remind you every day.

Do it now.

Record your actions every day. Completing the diary will help you build a brain-healthy habit.

1

Invest in Brain Health

"Every man can, if he so desires, become the sculptor of his own brain."
Santiago Ramón y Cajal

We all brush our teeth every day but most of us never spare a thought for our brains.

How crazy is that?

Of course, dental health is super important because you need your teeth to eat, to speak, and to smile. But you need your brain for everything, and I mean everything. There isn't one thing that you can do without your brain. You can't read this book, you can't turn this page, and you can't sit down or stand up without your brain. Come to think of it, you can't even brush your teeth without your brain.

You need your brain for everything, so brain health matters.

Why is brain health a smart investment?

You were obviously a smart kid because you grasped the complex concept of investment at a very young age. Time spent now brushing your teeth reaps future benefits. You developed a dental-health habit that includes daily brushing because you understood that that investment extends the life of your teeth and protects against tooth decay and dental pain in the future. You know that other activities like flossing, dental visits, and diet offer further protection.

However, as a grown-up you come to understand that even if you fastidiously follow your dentist's advice, your investment doesn't come with an absolute guarantee, but rather reduces the risk of pain and delays the onset of decay. Chances are, by the time you reach my age you will have had a couple of fillings and may even need some major work on a crumbling tooth or two. Nonetheless, you know that your teeth are in far better shape than they would have been without daily brushing.

The same applies to brain health.

Certain activities offer protection against decline in brain functions in later life, while some lifestyle choices increase your risk of developing diseases that affect brain function, such as Alzheimer's disease and other dementias. The important take-home message is that key lifestyle changes and activities that reduce risk or offer protection can easily be incorporated into your daily routine.

As is the case with dental health, having a good brain-health habit is not an absolute guarantee but there is plenty of evidence to suggest that it is definitely a worthwhile investment, especially if you fancy holding on to important cognitive functions such as memory for as long as possible. Maintaining and optimizing brain health will allow you to maximize your overall ability and independence.

Your brain is unique

Your brain allows you to think, to feel, to plan, to love, to laugh, to remember, and lots more besides. But that's not all; your brain also controls your senses and other parts of your body, including your muscles, organs, and blood vessels. Despite this brilliance you carry it around in your skull without giving it a second thought.

Scientists used to think that the brain was fixed, set like concrete, but we now know that the brain is constantly changing, sculpted by behaviors, experiences, and life choices. One of the big things you can do to help your brain is to adopt a brain-healthy lifestyle.

Your brain is unique, crafted by the experiences that you offer it and the demands that you place on it each and every day. Your brain is a dynamic organ that not only influences your behavior but is also influenced *by* your behavior. What you do or don't do influences how well your brain functions now and how resilient it can be when faced with future challenges. Your brain is constantly changing and it is your behaviors and your experiences that shape it.

Your brain is plastic—not credit-card plastic but pliable like putty. This neuroplasticity is a fundamental feature of the human brain. It's not exclusive to humans but the human brain does appear to excel at adaptation. While genetics[7] determine brain size in humans and chimpanzees, the human brain is more responsive to environmental influences, allowing it and its behavior to constantly adapt to changes. We tend to afford a lot of importance to our genes, but lifestyle and life experiences are critical to determining the shape of the brain, how it grows, and how it evolves. You can change your brain through experience. Learning can shape it rather like exercising can shape your muscles.

Accumulate information

When it comes to improving your finances, one of the best steps you can take is to improve your financial knowledge. You could do this by acquiring an understanding of financial concepts and risks as well as opportunities for investment. Gaining knowledge about yourself and your current finances and assets will also help inform your financial decisions and help maximize the return on any investment that you make. A good investment plan will acknowledge your unique needs, allowing you to live well now, plan for your future, and have choice and resilience built in should times get tough.

The same applies to improving your brain health. By reading this book you are taking a very important first step by increasing your knowledge of neuroscience, of dementia risk, and of opportunities for investment in brain health. By completing the questionnaires and diaries throughout the book, you will accumulate important information about yourself, your current habits, your assets and risks. This personal information will help to inform your choices and decisions to bring focus to your investment in brain health, while helping to minimize dementia risk and maximize the return on your investment. In this book you will pull together all of that information to create an honest and personal Brain Health Profile that will inform your initial plan and your longer-term brain-health investment strategy.

Diversify

Your Brain Health Profile is a bit like a financial portfolio. Good financial advice recommends diversification to help manage risk. There is no "one-size-fits-all" approach to financial investment. Advisers recommend creating an investment mix based on your financial goals, current financial situation, the timeline you are working within, and the amount of risk you can tolerate. They encourage diversity among and within different types of stocks, bonds, and other investments. Diversification doesn't come with any guarantee of success, but the investment mix allows you to potentially offset some of the impact if one aspect of your portfolio declines or performs poorly.

The recommendation for diversification also applies to brain health. A "one-size-fits-all" plan won't wash for brain health either. You need to create a brain-health investment mix that is based on your personal goals, your current brain-health situation, the timeline that you are working within (your age, your life stage), and the amount of risk factors that you have and can modify. I encourage diversity among and within different types of brain-healthy investment categories, too. In addition to building a mix of investments across sleep, stress management, social engagement, mental stimulation, heart health, physical activity, and attitude, you also need to have variety within these investments. For example, within physical activity you need to exercise aerobically, strengthen muscles, work on balance, and sit less.

Investing widely is investing wisely

Brain-health investment doesn't come with a guarantee that you won't develop dementia but it may help to defy it by offsetting some of the impact that the disease can have on your memory and your ability to sustain an independent life. While there are no guarantees when it comes to dementia in the broader sense, your return on brain-health investment will be handsome, rewarding you in multiple ways across your life. Through daily brain-healthy choices you will gain a sense of rejuvenation and greater satisfaction with life. You will also enjoy individual payoffs and fringe benefits in each of your investment categories, including better heart health, sounder sleep, more laughter, and sharper thinking and memory. When it comes to brain health, investing widely is investing wisely.

Regular check-ups

Financial advisers will also recommend giving your portfolio a regular check-up, at the very minimum once a year or any time your financial circumstances change significantly—such as if you lose your job or gain an inheritance. Regularly checking and updating your Brain Health Profile is also sound advice. Brain health is a long-term investment.

The Brain Health Plan that this book will help you to develop is the first step in a long-term strategy that aims to improve your brain health one day at a time. Regularly revisiting and updating your Brain Health Profile and Brain Health Plan will allow you to track your progress, take account of changing circumstances, and let you see whether you need to rebalance your "asset" mix or reconsider some of your individual investments.

Nothing to lose and everything to gain

Over the course of the next 100 days you will identify your brain-healthy habits and any behaviors that need fixing because they may be barriers to brain health or risk factors for dementia. You have nothing to lose and everything to gain. When it comes to brain health it is entirely within your power to transform your debts into assets by making conscious brain-healthy choices and simple changes to your daily life.

Brain health is for everyone

Whether you are embarking on retirement, are a student starting out in life, or at some point in between, this book aims to convince you to invest in brain health now. You possess an amazing resource inside your head: your brain is more complex than anything money can buy. Your brain is invaluable. It is the greatest gift you will ever receive, so treasure it, nurture it, and stimulate it so that you can reach your full potential throughout your entire life.

It's never too early or too late to invest in brain health.

Everyone with a brain needs to consider brain health.

Take action now

Your brain is shrinking. From our thirties onwards we lose a little brain volume[8] each year through a process called "atrophy"; hit sixty and the rate of that atrophy accelerates. But all is not lost, this book explains how living a brain-healthy life may help you to counteract atrophy and maintain brain volume.

The life choices that we make and the experiences that we have, even as children, can increase our risk of developing diseases that impair cognitive function in later life. Like most late-life disorders, the determinants of Alzheimer's disease and other dementias stretch right back across the lifespan. The following chapters explain that many of these determinants are modifiable, which means that you can take action now to reduce risk later.

Even a child's brain will struggle to develop normally in the absence of a stimulating, nurturing, brain-healthy environment. The experiences that we have in early life and those that we give our children impact on their brain health and brain development, affecting not only how their brain functions in childhood but how well it serves them across their entire lives.

The teenage brain goes through a dramatic period of neural reorganization. Neuronal networks[9] strengthen with use and unused networks are pruned as the brain matures. Teenage years can be a stressful time and parts of the brain involved in memory function are particularly vulnerable to stress. Adolescence represents an opportune time to condition healthy functioning of this part of the brain through brain-healthy life choices that have the potential for long-lasting positive impact.

A sense of invincibility may blind young adults to the need to invest in their future selves. The earlier the investment in brain health begins, the bigger the rewards. While protection against late-life diseases may not be a priority or even make the radar of young adults, none of us can predict whether we might sustain a brain injury in an accident or while playing sport. Healthier brains are more resilient and have a better chance of bouncing back from or compensating for such setbacks. The time to think about brain health is now.

Even if you have been in possession of a brain for more than sixty years, it will continue to change. The traditional adage is, quite frankly, wrong—you *can* teach an old dog new tricks. Living a brain-healthy life that is challenging and engaged is critical for cognitive function, especially as we now clock up more years than our ancestors. The quality of those extra years can be enhanced through brain-healthy choices.

Investing in brain health will cost you nothing but time and effort. The brain-healthy recommendations in this book can all be followed for free. That doesn't mean that they are easy, although some are, but they are within your control and can be integrated into your daily life.

Prevent and optimize

When we asked people across Europe what they feared most about growing old they answered—losing their memory and their independence. They also said that dementia was the disease that they feared most. Sadly, their fears aren't unfounded. While people are living longer, failing mental function frequently impairs the quality of those extra years. Cognitive decline has emerged as one of the greatest health threats of later life.

Failing mental function is the single biggest obstacle to independent living and to the social integration of older people. Cognitive impairment that does not reach the threshold for dementia diagnosis is not only associated with increased risk for progression to dementia, but also increased health-care costs, neuropsychiatric symptoms, and disability.

Brain health is not just about prevention, it is also about optimization. Living a brain-healthy life will not only help reduce dementia risk and maintain memory function in the future, but will also optimize brain performance in the here and now, enhancing the quality of your life today. Even if you already have a diagnosis or are experiencing memory impairment, making brain-healthy choices will help to optimize your brain function.

Aging and dementia

Differences in cognitive performance in people of different ages, with decline reported for older people, are well documented. Traditionally when there is no disease present in the brain these age-associated cognitive deficits have been considered a consequence of the aging process. However, the assumption that cognitive decline is inevitable can be questioned when you consider that a) a significant proportion of older adults do not demon-strate this decline and b) we see considerable differences across older adults in terms of the nature and the severity of cognitive disturbances that are evident in those experiencing cognitive decline.

There are close to fifty million people living with dementia in the world today. That figure is set to double every twenty years, reaching approx-imately 132 million by 2050. These predictions and the absence of a cure make prevention imperative. The global cost of dementia in 2018 is about one trillion U.S. dollars. A figure set to rise to two trillion by 2030.

One new case of dementia is diagnosed every three seconds.

The good news

My mom was one of those cases. I feel for anyone who receives a diagnosis because I understand the life-changing impact of dementia for the individual and for those who love them. Thankfully, the scientific evidence on dementia risk reduction is evolving rapidly. The identification of actionable risk factors that have the capacity to protect individuals from the onset and progression of dementia symptoms represents a wonderful opportunity to change the future—for ourselves, for our children, and for our grandchildren.

The World Health Organization prioritizes prevention and acknowl-edges that evidence is now sufficient to justify action to incorporate dementia risk reduction into health policies. *Up to half of all cases of Alzheimer's disease are attributable to just seven modifiable risk factors:*

- Physical inactivity
- Cognitive inactivity/low educational attainment
- Poorly managed hypertension (high blood pressure)
- Type 2 diabetes
- Mid-life obesity
- Smoking
- Depression

Taking account of the fact that many of these risk factors are inter-linked (such as obesity, physical inactivity, diabetes) about 30 percent of cases in Europe, UK, and the United States are attributable to these seven lifestyle factors.

We know that prevention is a legitimate evidence-based approach and the time has come to move from a singular focus on treatment and management of the disease to a focus that prioritizes dementia prevention and brain health. Reducing the prevalence of these seven risk factors by just 10 percent per decade would reduce the prevalence of Alzheimer's disease in 2050 by 8.3 percent globally.

Chapters 3 to 8 explain why each key lifestyle factor included in the program is critical for brain health. By completing the assessments in these chapters you will build a personal profile that will give you a clear picture of your assets and risks for each factor, allowing you to identify personal goals to address any barriers to brain health. The down-to-earth tips in each chapter will help you to devise a practical step-by-step action plan to increase your assets and reduce your risks for each factor.

Completing the 100-Day Diary at the end of this book forms an integral part of your action plan. Doing at least one thing every day is key to building a brain-healthy habit. Recording the actions that you take each day in your diary will help to keep you on track.

Chances are you are already doing lots of things every day that are good for your brain health. It's just as important to celebrate these healthy habits in your 100-Day Diary and on social media, if you've decided to share your journey with friends and family online.

The important thing is to make a conscious effort to make every day a brain-healthy day.

The false belief that dementia is a normal part of aging is still widely held. The program in this book is built on scientific research that shows that simple lifestyle changes and even some attitude adjustments can boost brain health and act as a buffer against decline in brain function. The next chapter shares the good news that your brain is resilient. Read on to learn how you can build reserves to boost your brain health.

2

Bank Reserves

"We are what we repeatedly do. Excellence then, is not an act, but a habit."
Aristotle

When a hard time hits, it helps to have something in reserve. In an economic recession, savings can get you through a tough patch. In nature, animals that hibernate stock up on stored energy that they can draw on over winter. Our brains can also have reserves, which can be drawn upon in the face of aging, damage, and disease. To explain this phenomenon a distinction is sometimes made between brain reserve and cognitive reserve.

One way of thinking about this slightly artificial distinction is that the brain reserve is the hardware and the cognitive reserve is the software. Our lifetime exposures—including our education, our jobs, and our leisure activities—can allow us to maintain our brain reserves and increase cognitive reserve. This is a very active area of research and the concept of reserve continues to evolve as the mysteries of the brain are revealed.

Atrophy refers to the wasting away of any part of the body. Your brain can atrophy by about 2 percent every ten years, leading to less brain and a loss of function. Brain atrophy, also called cerebral atrophy, describes the loss of brain cells and the connections between them. It can happen in just one part of the brain or it can occur across the entire brain. It all sounds a bit gloomy, but don't despair because brain atrophy is linked to many preventable, modifiable, and reversible factors.

Adopting a brain-healthy approach to life that excludes smoking and includes regular physical exercise, social engagement, and mental stimulation, together with a healthy diet and optimal amounts of sleep and stress, may help to prevent or slow down the rate at which your brain shrinks. The brief assessments in this chapter are repeated again at the end of the 100 days so that you can compare your scores pre- and post-program. Read on to learn how reserve works, why you need it, and how you can you bank it.

Brain Gains: What Is Reserve?

The idea that the brain can be resilient in the face of disease, aging, and even injury stems from the repeated observation that there is no direct relationship between the degree of brain disease or injury and the clinical manifestations of that disease or injury. Essentially, clinicians repeatedly noticed that the severity of damage or disease in the brain is not always related to the severity of symptoms.

For example, a head injury of the same magnitude can result in completely different levels of cognitive impairment and different recovery trajectories in different patients. Similarly, a stroke of the same size can produce profound effects on cognitive function in one patient and milder effects in another.

Some people also seem to be able to tolerate more age-related brain changes and even Alzheimer's disease-related pathology than others while still maintaining cognitive function. In the introduction to this book I mentioned that up to a quarter of people who have sufficient pathology in their brain post-mortem for a diagnosis of Alzheimer's disease do not show any cognitive impairment prior to death. The concept of reserve is used to account for this resilience.

BRAIN BASICS

The inner workings of the brain revealed by modern technology and scientific advancement offer us a mere glimpse of the brain's glorious magnificence. There is so much more to learn but for now we know enough to understand that the brain is a dynamic organ that not only influences our behavior but is also influenced *by* our behavior.

Evolved

According to one theory, three distinct brains emerged successively over time to become the complex interconnected organ that inhabits your skull today. Working from the inside out, the core—the oldest part in evolutionary terms—contains the brain stem, the stalk that connects your brain to your spinal cord. The stalk-like brain stem contains structures that control life-supporting functions that you don't have to consciously think about, such as heart rate, blood pressure, breathing, and digestion.

The second "brain," known as the limbic brain, first emerged in small mammals about 150 million years ago and it is thought that it evolved to manage "fight or flight" circuitry. You will read a lot about its main structures—the hippocampus and the amygdala—in this book because they are involved in learning, memory, emotions, mood, fear, stress, and the unconscious judgments that can strongly influence your behavior.

The hippocampus, which is shaped like a seahorse, is one of the most studied areas of the brain. It is particularly vulnerable to damage in Alzheimer's disease but is also an area of the brain capable of actually growing new neurons (neurogenesis) right across the lifespan. Your almond-shaped amygdala, located at the end of the hippocampus, is an important component of the limbic system, playing a key role in social behavior and in the processing and memory of emotional reactions—particularly within the context of fear.

The "third brain," the neocortex, as the name suggests, is a relative newcomer in the evolution of the brain, emerging in primates only two or three million years ago as the genus Homo emerged. It is part of the cerebral cortex[10] and is responsible for all of the higher-order functions that we associate with being human. By that I mean that it is involved in complex functions such as language and thought as well as sensory perception and the generation of motor commands. What is fascinating about the neocortex is that it is flexible and appears to have an infinite capacity to make learning happen.

Convoluted

The brain is divided into left and right cerebral hemispheres. The ridges and grooves that give the brain's outer cortex its convoluted, crinkly appearance are an ingenious exercise in Ikea-style space saving that allows more brain to fit inside your skull. *The human brain would take up approximately one square meter if you were to iron out all those wrinkles and lay it flat in your living room.*

Human cognition is complex. To make it easier to understand cognitive functioning we talk about six key neurocognitive domains. They are: learning and memory, executive function, complex attention, social cognition, language, and perceptual-motor function.

When it comes to these cognitive functions the work of the brain is, broadly speaking, split up among different sections of the crinkly cerebral cortex. Scientists divide the cortex into lobes, which are anatomical regions that are associated with certain processes. These four lobes are not stand-alone organs; they interact with each other and with the rest of your brain. Each lobe depends on information from other parts of the brain and from the world around you to get the job of being you done.

The frontal lobes, which sit just behind your forehead, play a key role in many of the executive functions that allow you to integrate information from other parts of your brain and from your environment so that you can make plans, think critically, solve problems, pay attention, make decisions, control your impulses, and understand and anticipate the consequences of your own behaviors.

The parietal lobes that lie behind the frontal lobes process information coming in from the various senses and link this with your memories and meaning.

The occipital lobes are located at the back of your head, behind the parietal lobes and just above the cerebellum (the little brain), which looks a bit like a tennis ball and sits just above the nape of your neck. Your occipital lobes are literally the eyes in the back of your head, because this part of the brain processes visual information.

The temporal lobes, which run along the sides of your head, are involved in processing sound. This includes perceiving sound, assigning meaning to sounds, remembering sounds, decoding auditory information—including distinguishing the volume and frequency of sounds—as well as understanding language and producing speech.

While everyone's lobes follow a similar structure, your personal-life exposures mean that your lobes will be unique to you because your life experiences continually bend and shape your brain.

Talking heads

Your brain contains billions of interconnected cells that "talk" to each other so that you can sense the sun on your face, chat with friends, anticipate your holidays, dread your exams, learn how to use your new phone, remember where you parked your car, decide what clothes to wear, or think about politics, philosophy, or instant noodles.

Your brain is made up of approximately 86 billion neurons, according to Brazilian neuroscientist Suzana Herculano-Houzel, who used a clever method that involved making "brain soup" to count them. Each and every one of these neurons forms an average of seven to ten thousand connections with other neurons, which means there are as many neuronal connections in your brain as there are stars in the Milky Way.

Neurons, also known as neurones and nerve cells, are the basic working unit of the brain. Their main function is to transmit information. In fact, communication between these nerve cells forms the basis of all brain function. Every time you make a movement, feel the wind in your face, hear a voice, or recall a memory, that information is moving along and between neurons through an electro-chemical process.

Neurons typically have highly specialized extensions coming out of the cell body. The branch-like dendrite acts like an aerial that receives incoming information and relays it to the neuron's cell body, which acts like mission control. Cable-like extensions called axons carry information away from mission control to other neurons in your brain and to other types of cells in your body.

In the cell body, all of the incoming signals are added together and a response signal is generated where the cell meets its axon. The electrical signal is sent along the axon to the nerve terminal where it is converted to a chemical signal. The point where the axon of one neuron connects with the dendrite of another is called a synapse, which is a physical gap between neurons where information from one neuron transfers to another. Synapses release chemical messengers called neurotransmitters. You have between 100 and 500 trillion synapses.

Pathways

The route that a piece of information takes through neurons around your brain is called a pathway, and the more you use a pathway the more defined it gets. A bit like a well-trodden track through a field or forest. When you learn something new—take up a sport, walk a new route to work, learn a new language, or learn how to resist decadent desserts, it can seem challenging at first. But as you repeat tasks you forge or "wire" stronger pathways in your brain and over time the new tasks become second nature. Remember this as you try to introduce new brain-healthy habits.

In addition to neurons, your brain contains billions of glial cells that play a critical role in keeping your brain working healthily. If the neurons in your brain are like information highways, glial cells are the builders— the fixers, the protectors, and the service providers—that help to keep your electro-chemical neuron show on the road, 24/7. Neurons need to send nerve impulses rapidly. Glial cells help neurons to do this by wrapping themselves around the axon to form an insulation sheath (like the insulation around electrical wires in your home). The sheath, which is made up of a white fatty substance called myelin, accelerates neural conduction.

The portions of the brain that contain myelinated nerve fibers are commonly referred to as white matter, due to the color of myelin. In contrast, gray matter contains the neural cell bodies, dendrites, and axon terminals.

RESERVE

In essence, reserve is a way of explaining the disconnection between the degree of brain damage or disease and the clinical expression of that damage or disease, including the impact it has on cognitive function.

Brain reserve

Brain reserve is the structural stuff: gray matter, white matter, and the thickness of the cortex. Brain reserve refers to the actual differences in the brain itself that might explain how one individual has greater tolerance to damage than another.

Size matters

Let's take Mary and Jane, for example. Both have the same amount of plaques and tangles in their brains but their brains are different sizes. Mary has more neurons, greater synaptic density, and a larger brain than Jane. This means that Mary has more brain without disease than Jane has. Mary, with the larger brain, will be more resilient than Jane to the effects of the same amount of disease pathology. It is not the amount of disease in the brain that accounts for differences in cognitive functioning between people, it is the amount of intact brain.

When you compare people with different levels of cognitive function you find that these differences are related to the size of the individual's brain rather than to the amount of disease within it. To put it simply: brain size matters.

An individual might not show impairment in cognitive functioning because they have more neurons and more synapses to lose before they reach the critical threshold at which clinical symptoms will appear. As the disease progresses, the amount of diseased brain will increase and the amount of intact brain will decrease until a certain point is reached where the intact brain can no longer maintain normal cognitive functioning.

Brain reserve means that the brain's structural characteristics provide resilience against the atrophy or wasting associated with aging or disease. The larger your adult brain is, the longer you can resist the impact of damage or disease on your functioning.

Brain maintenance

At any given point in time you have a certain amount of brain reserve, and the higher your brain reserve the better you will do in the face of brain changes caused by aging, injury, or disease. We used to think that once these brain reserves were depleted that was it, they were gone and you would succumb to clinical symptoms or deficits, just like we used to think that once you reached adulthood you had a certain amount of neurons and all you could do from that point on was lose them.

However, we now know that brain reserve is more nuanced. We know that your brain changes with experience. Stimulating environments can lead to the growth of new neurons. Brain-derived neurotropic factor (BDNF), dubbed "Miracle-Gro for the brain," is a molecule[11] that plays a key role in neuroplasticity, improves neuronal function, protects cells from stress and cell death, and encourages neurons to grow, just as fertilizer encourages plants to grow. BDNF is vital for learning, and the good news is that aerobic exercise is associated with increased BDNF concentration and enhanced cognitive function. Stimulating environments also lead to increased levels of BDNF, promoting neuroplasticity.

The latest thinking is that it *is* possible to maintain your brain reserves. Your brain will atrophy as you age but you can counteract this wasting by engaging in activities that promote neurogenesis and neuroplasticity.

Think for a moment about all of the retired people that you have ever known. I'd hazard a guess that if you are thinking of ten retirees aged over sixty-five, one may have developed Alzheimer's disease while one or two have remained as sharp as a razor. The rest fall somewhere in between, a little slower at processing information than they used to be, they might also be having some trouble remembering new stuff but almost all of them have retained the ability to regale you with stories from their youth. Truth be told, you've heard the stories so many times you could probably tell them yourself. The reality is that while many individuals do experience decline in later life there is no real consistency with regard to the nature or the severity of the disturbances that people experience to their cognitive functioning.

A relative lack of brain pathology is the biggest contributor to this diversity in cognitive functioning. Of course, the less pathology you have the better, but it does also seem that various lifestyle factors can contribute to resisting the effects of disease-induced pathology and the advent of age-related brain changes.

Brain maintenance contributes to your current levels of brain reserves. Certain activities—for example, mental stimulation (Chapter

5) and physical exercise (Chapter 7)—are actually linked with changes in the brain itself. Increased cognitive activity may help to preserve the volume of your whole brain and particularly the volume of the hippocampus, the part of your brain involved in memory and learning. Physical exercise has also been linked with increased total brain and hippocampal volume. Some people maintain their brains (and brain reserves) more successfully than others and this phenomenon may be down to differences in exposure to particular life experiences such as education, occupations, and certain leisure activities. After all, the brain is plastic, which is a fancy way of saying that it can change itself in response to experience and learning.

Cognitive reserve

Cognitive reserve refers to the plasticity or flexibility of cognitive networks in the face of disruption caused by aging, injury, or disease. Let's consider Ben and Kim, who have the same amount of hardware (brain reserve). Ben can tolerate more age-related brain changes because the capacity of his underlying software (cognitive reserve) differs from Kim's in a way that allows his brain to cope with or adapt to the disruptions.

So with cognitive reserve it is how the brain functions rather than structural brain size that differs across people and explains the disconnect between pathology or other types of brain change and the clinical manifestation of the disease or brain change. *In the context of Alzheimer's disease, cognitive reserve describes the capacity of an adult brain to sustain Alzheimer's disease pathology without manifesting clinical symptoms of dementia at a level that would be sufficient to cause clinical dementia in an individual with less cognitive reserve.*

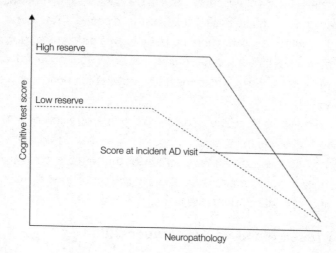

Figure 1: This illustration demonstrates how cognitive function might change over time in two individuals, one with high reserve and one with low reserve. The Alzheimer's disease pathology begins to advance in the brain of both individuals before any changes are observed. At some point the pathology will be sufficient to cause changes. These changes can be measured on cognitive tests. You will see that the point where performance begins to decline occurs later in the individual with high reserve. They can tolerate more disease pathology before it affects their cognitive performance. Eventually there will be a point where performance is the same for both, but that point occurs much later in the disease process for the individual with high reserve. Once decline begins in the individual with high reserve it will occur rapidly. This model explains the different trajectories of decline we often see in individuals with Alzheimer's disease.

Illustration from Stern, Y. (2012), "Cognitive reserve in aging and Alzheimer's disease," *The Lancet.*

Tolerance

A key assumption underlying cognitive reserve is that Alzheimer's disease slowly develops over time, so that the pathology is present in the brain for several years before the disease is clinically diagnosed. People with higher cognitive reserve tolerate more disease pathology than people with lower cognitive reserve before symptoms appear, so that the onset of the clinical dementia will be delayed.

However, you will remember from my example of Peter and Jake on page 3 that once people with higher cognitive reserve start to show cognitive changes they tend to have more rapid progression of their dementia symptoms. In essence, this is because their symptoms have appeared much later in the course of the disease. They begin their outward cognitive decline when the pathology is much more advanced in the brain, so they have less time between the onset of clinical symptoms and the point where the pathology in their brain overwhelms their function.

On a positive note, if you consider the entire duration of time they have had the Alzheimer's disease pathology in their brain, the upside is that they spend a greater proportion of that time in possession of their cognitive faculties and a smaller proportion of their life with their functioning devastated by this disease.

Neural reserve and neural compensation

There are two facets to cognitive reserve: neural reserve and neural compensation.

When you compare two people with normal healthy brains, the cognitive processing in their brains won't be identical; they will be different from each other. Neural reserve reflects this difference in cognitive processing across people.

Neural compensation, on the other hand, refers to changes in cognitive processing that may occur to cope with brain pathology, with other types of brain changes, or even when tasks that we engage in become increasingly more challenging.

Neural reserve reflects differences in the brain networks that underlie cognitive performance. Again thinking about the software analogy, it may be the case that a person whose neural networks are more efficient, more flexible, or have greater capacity is better able to cope when the system is disrupted by disease.

Depending on the task at hand, because of our unique life experiences, my neural processing of a task might be less efficient than your neural processing of the same task. For example, if disease strikes both of us, the superior efficiency of your networks might allow you to carry out the task (i.e., find the word that you need) while my less-efficient processing might mean that when faced with disease disruption my network can no longer process the task and a deficit emerges (i.e., I can't find the right word).

Neural compensation reflects the differences in people's ability to recruit alternative networks in their brain when their standard processing networks have been disrupted by disease, injury, or aging. Rather than doing nothing when the brain is challenged or when pathology threatens the brain's integrity, the brain actively tries to continue to do its job and copes with damage by employing neural networks and using brain structures not normally used by individuals with intact brains for the particular task at hand.

Work

In the early days of reserve research, scientists found that individuals with less than eight years of education were more than twice as likely to develop dementia compared to those with more education. They wondered whether mentally stimulating jobs might also have the capacity to boost reserves. They grouped people taking part in their research according to what they described as low occupational attainment (unskilled/semi-skilled, skilled trade/craft, and clerical/office worker) or high occupational attainment (business manager/government and professional/technical).

They found that those with low lifetime occupational attainment were also more than twice as likely to develop dementia than those with higher lifetime occupational attainment.

Leisure

Next they turned their attention to leisure activities, given that so many of these can be mentally stimulating, to see whether they might impart reserve against the expression of Alzheimer's pathology as clinical dementia. They interviewed a different group of older adults who did not have a diagnosis of Alzheimer's disease and asked them whether in the previous month they had taken part in any of the thirteen activities listed below:

- Knitting, music, or other hobby
- Walking for pleasure or excursion
- Visiting friends or relatives
- Being visited by friends or relatives
- Physical conditioning

- Going to movies, restaurants, or sports events
- Reading magazines, newspapers, or books
- Watching television or listening to the radio
- Doing unpaid community volunteer work
- Playing cards, games, or bingo
- Going to a club or center
- Going to classes
- Going to church or synagogue or temple

When they divided the participants according to low (less than six) and high (more than six) leisure-activity participation they found that those who engaged in more leisure activities had less risk of developing dementia. From the findings of more than twenty studies that look at the effects of education, occupation, and engaging in mentally stimulating activities on incident dementia, it is estimated that the protective effect of cognitive reserve inferred by these activities reduces the risk of developing dementia by 46 percent.

> **No-Brainer**: Engage in stimulating activities to maintain your brain reserves and increase cognitive reserve. Repeating brain-healthy habits will eventually override old patterns of behavior.

Brain Drains: What Happens in Your Brain When You Age?

With age the overall size of your brain shrinks. The molecules, cells, and blood vessels in the brain can also change, impacting your cognitive function. There is an overall atrophy (shrinkage) of the entire brain. The brain also shrinks from the inside out because the cavities (ventricles[12]) within your brain become enlarged. In some regions of the brain there is a loss of neurons, a deterioration of dendrites (branches) and axons (cables), and a decrease in neurotransmitters (chemical messengers).

There is also a regional decline in blood flow and the rate at which energy is expended (metabolic rate). Aging can also be associated with the appearance of abnormal clusters of the chemically "sticky" proteins in gray matter called plaques, as well as twisted fibers of protein called tangles. These plaques are seen in the frontal and temporal lobes in typical aging, in contrast to Alzheimer's disease where the plaques are found predominantly in the hippocampus and the locus coeruleus,[13] both of which are involved in learning and memory.

Your brain is shrinking

Brain volume reduction begins early in life and continues at a gradual pace throughout adulthood. By the time you hit thirty, significant shrinkage has already occurred. A large part of the reduction in overall brain volume across your lifespan will be due to reductions in gray matter volume.

Volume

For most of your adult life you will lose about 0.2 percent of brain volume each year. In the later part of your life that rate of volume loss increases to just under 0.5 percent per year. In Alzheimer's disease the rate of volume loss is doubled compared to people the same age who don't have a diagnosis of Alzheimer's.

On average, between the ages of thirty and ninety you can expect to lose a third of your hippocampus, a quarter of your cerebral white matter and 14 percent of your cerebral cortex. Atrophy is not uniform across the cortex, so while your temporal, parietal, and occipital lobes reduce by about 1 percent, your prefrontal cortex[14] is pretty badly hit, with a 22 percent reduction in volume between your fifth and seventh decades, and a whopping 43 percent reduction to coincide with retirement at sixty-five.

White matter

While we know that white matter changes with aging, the reason for these changes is unclear, but it may be related to the age-related slowing of information-processing in the brain. White matter has highly organized tracts. Poor executive function and poor verbal fluency are related to deterioration of the white matter tracts in the aging brain, especially in the frontal regions of the brain.

If your executive functioning was affected you might, for example, have difficulty managing time, maintaining focus, remembering details, paying attention, or resisting saying things. Verbal fluency is a cognitive function that depends on executive control and involves retrieving information from memory.

Assessment: Verbal Fluency

For this assessment you will need a timer and a voice recorder* (such as the voice memo app on your phone). Set a timer for one minute and record yourself naming as many animals you can in that time.

Your score is the total of admissible words—names of extinct, imaginary, or magical animals are admissible but given names for animals like "Spot" or "Fluffy" are not. Wrong words, variations, and repetitions are not counted as correct.

Listen back and record your total correct score ____

What your score means
Age and education influence how people perform on this task. Average scores are:
   Age 16–59:
         9–12 years of education = 20;
         13–21 years of education = 22.
   Age 60–79:
         0–8 years of education = 14;
         9–12 years of education = 16;
         13–21 years of education = 18.
   Age 80–95:
         0–8 years of education = 13;
         9–12 years of education = 14;
         13–21 years of education = 16.

The above will give you an indication of whether you are performing above, below, or within the average range for your age.

---

* If you don't have access to a voice recorder, ask a friend to count your admissible correct responses as you name the animals.

Atrophy linked to lifestyle

When it comes to neurons and synapses, the loss is also selective, with neurons lost in some brain regions and preserved in others. Generally speaking, in a typically aging brain, neurons are lost in the cerebral cortex in frontal and temporal regions, in the hippocampi (you have two, one in each hemisphere), in the brain stem, and in the locus coeruleus. These structural changes affect connectivity in the brain and functional responsiveness.

Research with animals shows that the cellular basis of learning and memory is more difficult to achieve in older animals than in younger animals. All this loss with age sounds a bit gloomy but the more we are learning about the aging brain the more we are coming to understand that even though brain shrinkage is progressive, brain atrophy can be slowed or even reversed through lifestyle changes. This makes perfect sense given that brain atrophy is closely related to cardiovascular disease, obesity, diabetes, poor sleep habits, and stress.

Slower but still accurate

The brain can remain relatively healthy and function well in later life. In fact, disease is the cause of most decline. In the absence of brain disease most people experience a general slowing in processing speed and some decline in the ability to form new memories for recent events as they age. But even at that, many instances that we describe as memory failures—such as forgetting where we left our keys—might actually be failures of attention rather than genuine memory failures. If you don't "attend" to where you put something you can't encode the memory of putting it there and it is very difficult to recall a memory that you never encoded.

Assessment: Memory, Health, and Well-Being

You will need a pen and paper to complete this task.

Read the following list for about thirty seconds, concentrating on each word for a few seconds only.

1a. Remember these words:

Cat	Piano	Carrot	Table
Window	Bread	Summer	Hat
Grass	Van	Phone	Nail

1b. Now close the book and write down as many words as you can recall.

Your score is the total number of words that you recalled correctly.

Your score ____

What your score means

The average number of chunks of information that can be stored in short-term memory is seven—plus or minus two. If you scored between five and nine your short-term memory is working at an average capacity. If you scored more than nine or less than five then you are performing above or below average respectively.

2. **How would you rate your general health at the present time?**

   Excellent ☐   Very good ☐   Good ☐   Fair ☐   Poor ☐

3. **How would you rate your overall sense of well-being at the present time?**

   Excellent ☐   Very good ☐   Good ☐   Fair ☐   Poor ☐

4. **How would you rate your day-to-day memory at the present time?**

   Excellent ☐   Very good ☐   Good ☐   Fair ☐   Poor ☐

The effect of brain aging on cognitive function means that it requires more effort to remember what you wanted to buy at the supermarket, to process and respond to information and to reason your way through a problem. While it takes more time and effort, you can be consoled by the fact that your accuracy remains the same. It is also possible to compensate by practicing more. Vocabulary tends to remain, as do skills that have been practiced for a long time, and don't need to rely on processing speed. The good news is that some cognitive skills, such as knowledge and wisdom, may even improve with age.

Crystallized and fluid

We sometimes draw a distinction between "fluid" abilities and "crystallized" abilities. Crystallized ability reflects knowledge and experience that you have accumulated during your life. Fluid ability refers to your capacity to use that knowledge in an adaptable and flexible fashion.

Of course, these two aspects of your cognition are probably not independent because, for example, your current level of crystallized ability (knowledge and experience) may influence the effectiveness of your fluid abilities. The converse is also true, as your ability to accumulate knowledge may depend on your flexibility and adaptability.

Fluid abilities refer to faculties such as your ability to think and act quickly, solve new problems, and encode short-term memories. In contrast, crystallized abilities are reflected in tests of knowledge, general information, use of language, and a wide variety of acquired skills.

Fluid abilities appear to decline with age, while crystallized abilities tend to remain stable or even improve over the lifespan. Generally speaking, across the lifespan, crystallized abilities show a tendency to increase up to the sixth and seventh decades. It is only in late old age that decline, if any, emerges.

Aging and memory

In contrast, when it comes to memory function and processing speed there is a continuous linear decline during early adulthood, which then accelerates in later life.

Most cognitive changes reported with age are associated with memory and processing speed.

"It takes me longer to think a problem through."

"I forget where I left things."

"I can't remember names."

"It's on the tip of my tongue."

Our reaction time declines with age, too. As we get older we can become distracted more easily. In fact, aging is associated with difficulty suppressing the influence of irrelevant information, which can make it hard for us to be selective about the information we want to remember or pay attention to.

Older people consistently take longer on timed tasks than younger people, but their accuracy is the same. Speed of retrieval is affected, so finding the right name or word takes longer than it used to. The decline in processing speed actually begins when you are in your early thirties. Working memory ability, for example your ability to do mental arithmetic, decreases with age. Knowledge, memory for facts, and memory for procedures stay the same or even improve as we age.

When should I be concerned about my memory?

Forgetting where you put your keys for the third time in a week is not necessarily something that you need to see your doctor about. Nor is forgetting the name or face of a person that you just met or even someone that you haven't seen in years. However, if you, or someone you love:

- Get disoriented about where you are, or what time of day it is;
- Get lost in a place you've been familiar with for years;
- Start repeating the same story every day without realizing it;
- Experience problems that interfere with your life at home or at work or affect your/their quality of life;

it might be worth chatting to your doctor.

It can be frustrating not being able to find the right word, or to struggle to speak as fast as you would like to. When this happens, ban stress. If you feel stress welling up, try to stay calm, relax, take a deep breath and give your brain the time and the space that it needs to do what you want it to do. Give yourself permission to take as long as you need and don't be afraid to ask others to give you the time that you need. Everything doesn't have to happen at breakneck speed.

Chat to your doctor if you suspect that any prescribed medication is interfering with your cognitive functioning and discuss alternative options. Stay connected, especially during times of emotional upheaval or when you are feeling anxious or down. Seek the support of those who love you—sometimes simply voicing fears can give you perspective and may even help you to find solutions.

Pay heed to what those who love you are saying, too. They may notice problems before you do. Try to listen calmly and remember that they have your best interests at heart. It's never easy to hear these things but it's not easy for them to say them either. It can be helpful to discuss how you might manage such issues before there is a problem. If you are feeling depressed, take action sooner rather than later and resist the temptation to withdraw. Instead, keep exercising, keep engaging with life, and keep smiling.

A deep depression can cloud your thinking and impair memory. If you have been depressed or have felt persistently sad for weeks or months, take action now, visit a health professional. If you have already taken this step and feel that your current treatment is not working, talk to your doctor about alternative approaches until you find one that works for you.

Be honest with yourself about your limitations and don't try to pretend that you're not having increasing difficulty in remembering faces, places, or where you left your car keys or what you were going to say next.

Once you've faced up to those limitations, be kind to yourself and don't allow yourself to feel as if you're mentally falling apart. Start taking steps to remedy those lapses in your memory, in the same way that you might try to lose weight if you've put on a few extra pounds, or adopt strategies to support any flagging functions.

If you have noticed worrying changes in your memory, don't jump to conclusions and immediately think that it is the start of dementia. In addition to depression and some medications there are many things that can easily be remedied that can interfere with memory, including vitamin B12 deficiency, thyroid problems, dehydration, a severe infection, menopause, poor sleep, stress, and smoking. Don't postpone talking to your doctor, you may find that there is a simple solution.

Dementia

Dementia is arguably the most feared disease of later life. Huge stigma still surrounds it and as a consequence some misunderstandings persist. So I think it is worth taking the time to outline some key facts.

Nine out of ten older people don't get dementia, and many people make it to their eighties and nineties without much memory decline.

Dementia is not a single disease, it is not a normal part of aging, it is caused by a number of brain diseases that can change the brain and disturb various functions within it, including learning, memory, thinking, language, judgment, comprehension, calculation, and understanding of time and place. Dementia is the consequence of these diseases.

Unfortunately, to confuse matters the word dementia is also used as an umbrella term to describe the various conditions and diseases that lead to the disturbed function known as dementia. About 1 percent of people aged over sixty will get dementia. However, the prevalence doubles every five years so that approximately 25 percent of people over eighty-five will succumb to the disease. Although dementia usually affects people later in life, younger people can get it too; if it occurs before the age of sixty-five it is referred to as early onset dementia. Dementia does not affect everyone in the same way.

Alzheimer's disease, the most common form of dementia, accounts for about 60–80 percent of all cases of the disease. As a consequence, the bulk of dementia research focuses on Alzheimer's disease. Current thinking is that it is a "proteinopathic" disease, which just means that it is caused by malformed proteins in the brain. These proteins—beta-amyloid and tau respectively—form plaques and tangles in the brain, but it's not entirely clear how this leads to loss of neurons. Atrophy can been seen on CT scans in the hippocampi, the cortex, and the limbic areas. As already mentioned, the presence of this Alzheimer's disease pathology in the brain—the plaques and tangles—does not necessarily mean that the individual will have dementia symptoms.

Alzheimer's affects more women than men. In contrast, vascular dementia affects more men than women. Vascular dementia is a relatively common form of dementia caused by a number of common conditions that damage the brain's blood vessels, affecting their ability to deliver the oxygen and nutrients that the brain needs to survive and to carry out its work effectively. Conditions that can lead to vascular dementia include stroke and other conditions that inflict long-term damage to the brain's blood vessels, including high blood pressure, hardening of the arteries, and diabetes. Other common forms of dementia are mixed dementia (a combination of Alzheimer's disease and vascular pathology in the brain) and Lewy body dementia, which refers to both dementia with Lewy bodies (abnormal deposits of a protein called alpha-synuclein) and the dementia that occurs with Parkinson's disease.

Age is the biggest risk factor for dementia. In addition to the seven potentially modifiable risk factors associated with cognitive decline or Alzheimer's disease that I mentioned in Chapter 1, diet and social isolation are also implicated. A poor diet that is high in fat and has low vegetable intake is also consistently associated with increased risk. Evidence to date suggests that social isolation is another risk factor.

The relationship between some of these risk factors and dementia is complicated. While obesity in mid-life is associated with significantly increased risk of dementia, being obese over the age of sixty-five is associated with a reduced dementia risk and being underweight in later life is associated with an increased risk. This may be because body mass index (BMI) can decline up to ten years before dementia symptoms become apparent.

It is not clear which way the association between social isolation and dementia works. Is it social isolation that leads to dementia or does dementia lead to social withdrawal? Either way, it is important to address social isolation due to its association with depression, heart disease, and other health issues that impact on brain health.

While there is no denying the association between depression and dementia, there is some conflicting evidence. Rather than being a risk factor it could be that depression in later life represents an early symptom of dementia, or it could be that both depression and dementia share common causes.

Head injury can also increase risk; people with Down's syndrome are at increased risk of developing dementia, and family history and genetics can play a role, too, but the risk is low compared to that associated with lifestyle factors. Since there is currently no cure for dementia, risk factors that can be modified represent an important opportunity to delay or prevent the onset of dementia symptoms. If we could push out the onset of Alzheimer's disease by two years we could prevent almost 23 million cases of the disease by 2050!

No-Brainer: Minimize your dementia risk factors.

Summary

- Adopting a brain-healthy approach to life that excludes smoking and includes regular physical exercise, social engagement, and mental stimulation, together with a healthy diet and optimal amounts of sleep and stress, may help to prevent or slow down the rate at which your brain shrinks.
- There is no direct relationship between the degree of brain disease or brain injury and the clinical symptoms of that brain disease or injury.
- At any given point in time you have a certain amount of brain reserve, and the higher your brain reserve the better you will do in the face of brain changes caused by aging, injury, or disease.
- Stimulating environments can lead to the growth of new neurons (neurogenesis) and lead to increased levels of BDNF (the Miracle-Gro fertilizer), which in turn promotes neuroplasticity in your brain.
- Increased cognitive activity may help to preserve the volume of your brain and particularly that of your hippocampus, which plays a crucial role in memory and learning.
- Physical exercise has been linked with increased total brain and hippocampal volume.
- People with higher cognitive reserve tolerate more disease pathology than people with lower cognitive reserve before symptoms appear, so that the onset of the clinical dementia will be delayed.
- People who engage in more leisure activities have less risk of developing dementia.
- On average, between the ages of thirty and ninety you can expect to lose a third of your hippocampus, a quarter of your cerebral white matter, and 14 percent of your cerebral cortex.

- Even though brain shrinkage is progressive as you age, brain atrophy can be slowed or even reversed through changes to your lifestyle.
- Your brain can remain relatively healthy and function well in later life.
- As you age you are likely to experience a general slowing in the speed with which you can process information and you will also experience some decline in your ability to form new memories for recent events.
- While it might take more time and effort to do cognitive tasks, you can be consoled by the fact that your accuracy remains the same.
- The good news is that some of your cognitive skills, such as knowledge and wisdom, may even improve with age.
- Dementia is not a normal part of aging.
- Nine out of ten older people do not get dementia.
- Minimize dementia risk factors—this program will help you to do just that.

Brain Changers: What You Can Do

The very first step you can take toward protecting your precious brain is to minimize the risk of head injury. The most common causes of head injury are vehicle accidents, falls, and firearms. A significant number of head injuries are sustained in sport.

TEN PRACTICAL TIPS TO PROTECT YOUR BRAIN

1. Always wear a seatbelt.
2. Drive safely, don't text and drive, don't drink and drive, and don't drive when you are drowsy or have had insufficient sleep.
3. Wear a properly fitting helmet when cycling, motorcycling, sledding, snowmobiling, skateboarding, or, when advised, playing contact sports.
4. Use lights and wear reflective clothing when cycling in the dark.

5. Follow health and safety guidelines at work. Wear a hard hat where appropriate and use ladders and scaffolding safely.

6. Don't stand on an unstable chair to change a lightbulb, use a stepladder instead. When carrying out DIY, use appropriate equipment and make sure ladders are stable.

7. Remove tripping hazards around the home, especially on stairways. Put a non-slip mat in the shower. Clean up any spillages as soon as they occur.

8. If you have young kids, make sure windows can't be opened by curious little hands. Move furniture away from windows to prevent inquisitive children climbing onto them and falling out of open windows.

9. There are no second chances with guns. If you own a firearm, rigidly adhere to the safe storage and use guidelines.

10. Keep up to date with the latest research and medical advice with regard to minimizing and treating concussions, which are frequently sustained in a variety of sports, including American football, rugby, soccer, horse-riding, boxing, and trampolining. Minimize risk of head injury, and if you are a parent make sure you balance the risk of head injury with the benefit of physical activity when considering sports for your children.

3

Cherish Sleep

"Sleep is the golden thread that ties our health and our bodies together."
Thomas Dekker

SLEEP—PART ONE

You don't need me to tell you that sleep is essential. You know only too well that if you don't get enough sleep you become irritable and you can't think straight—in fact, pretty much all you can think about is getting some sleep. You need sleep. Your brain needs sleep. Your body needs sleep. Sleep is fundamental not just for brain health but also for physical and mental health.

According to a recent large-scale survey in the United States, just two-thirds of us regularly get a healthy night's sleep. One in three of us are not getting sufficient sleep, placing ourselves at risk of numerous chronic health conditions, cancers, and even premature death. The number of people getting fewer than the recommended hours of sleep every night in industrialized countries has increased to such an extent since the 1980s that the World Health Organization has declared a sleep-loss epidemic.

We don't need to develop a fancy vaccine to tackle this particular epidemic. There are plenty of things that we can do to improve sleep health. In this chapter you will find practical tips to help you sleep more soundly. You will also keep a Sleep Log and complete assessments that will give you a clearer understanding of your current sleep patterns and help you to transform your sleep habit to benefit your brain health. You will use this information to create your personal sleep profile, set goals, and devise a sleep action plan in Part Two of this chapter.

First, let's delve into the neuroscience of sleep to discover why we sleep and find out what occurs in the brain during sleep and what happens when the brain is deprived of sleep.

Quick Question: Sleep

Estimate how many hours you sleep each night ____

Brain Gains: Why Do We Sleep?

Have you ever wondered why a good night's sleep clears your head and you wake up feeling refreshed? Well, it turns out that brain washing might, quite literally, be the answer.

Brain washing

Lulu Xie spent two years in a laboratory in the University of Rochester training mice to relax and fall asleep on a special kind of microscope that can show the movement of dye through living tissue. Her incredible patience was rewarded with evidence for what may be sleep's fundamental function: brain washing. To be more precise, the basic reason why we sleep may be to clear the brain of the toxic byproducts of metabolism that accumulate during wakefulness. Metabolism refers to the chemical processes that occur within your body that keep you alive.

Recent research claims that sleep has a critical function in metabolic homeostasis. Maintaining metabolic homeostasis just means that your body has to keep conditions optimal both inside and outside your cells so that the life-supporting chemical reactions of metabolism can occur. Essentially, your body needs to convert food to energy to run your cells and create the compounds that your cells need to function and survive. The byproducts of metabolism and cellular waste need to be disposed of.

Nature's body detox

Like industrial chemical processing plants, your body has a system built into its architecture that deals with the safe disposal of waste and toxic byproducts. In your body a system of vessels that runs alongside your veins and arteries performs this function. This lymphatic system eliminates metabolic byproducts, surplus fluids, waste, and toxins. A fluid called lymph is carried away from your tissues and eventually returned to your bloodstream via this system of lymphatic vessels. As lymph flows through your lymphatic vessels it passes through lymph nodes where bacteria, cancer cells, and other potentially toxic agents are filtered.

You'll be familiar with swollen lymph nodes in your neck or under your arm if you've ever had an infection. They do a really important job of containing the spread of infection, cancer cells, or toxins. Every day your lymph vessels transport up to four liters of purified lymph back into your bloodstream for circulation.

The lymphatic system covers your entire body like a net. The density of these vessels is usually proportional to the metabolic rate of the tissue it serves, much like a filtration system in a chemical plant would need to be in proportion to the work being done by the processing plant. Given that your brain uses more energy than any other organ in your body, you'd expect it to have a really dense network of lymphatic vessels capable of rapidly eliminating the metabolic byproducts released through the high metabolic activity of your busy brain cells.

The absence of a lymphatic system in the brain has really puzzled scientists, especially as neurons are highly vulnerable to toxic waste products. Recently, one of these curious scientists, Dr. Maiken Nedergaard, discovered a series of microscopic fluid-filled channels that surround blood vessels within the brains of mice, which she dubbed the "glymphatic system" because its waste elimination activities are managed by glial cells.

Stars that clean at night

Like a network of pipes in an industrial plant, the glymphatic system carries cerebrospinal fluid[15] (CSF) laden with waste. Ultimately this system in your brain transports the waste to the same central excretion and recycling sites used by the rest of your body. This means that local protein processing and degradation is avoided within the brain. This makes perfect sense since it takes toxic waste away from the brain, a vital but vulnerable organ. Very recently, some lymphatic vessels have been discovered in the brains of mice, which look like they might serve as a second step in the waste removal process by carrying waste from cerebrospinal fluid (CSF) into nearby lymph nodes.

Space invaders

In industrial plants and many other types of buildings, interstitial space is used to incorporate various building-service elements, including waste removal. The fluid-filled spaces that surround the cells of your brain tissue are also known as interstitial space—which comprises 20 percent of the total volume of your brain—and this is where the waste products secreted by your brain cells are flushed away, with the help of CSF.

The CSF seeps through the interstitial space among the brain cells and eventually gets pumped back into the bloodstream at the meninges, which are the protective membranes that surround your brain. The transport of fluid across membranes requires a lot of energy, so Nedergaard had a hunch that the brain would not be able to carry out waste removal *and* process the sensory information that bombards us while we are awake. Following up on this hunch, Lulu Xie invested two years in training mice to sleep on the microscope, trying to establish whether activity of the glymphatic system ramps up during sleep.

By tracking different-colored dyes through the brains of mice, Lulu discovered that large amounts of CSF flowed into the brain during sleep but not when the mice were awake. It turns out that during wakefulness the flow of CSF is restricted to the surface of the brain and is only 5 percent of the flow she measured when the mice were asleep. During sleep the brain gets a really deep clean as CSF flows deep into the brain tissue. This expansion of 60 percent during sleep results in a more efficient clearance of metabolites including beta-amyloid, which accumulates during waking and is implicated in Alzheimer's disease.

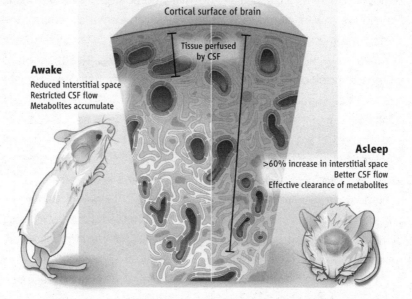

Figure 2: The extracellular (interstitial) space in the cortex of the mouse brain, through which cerebral spinal fluid moves, increases from 14% in the awake animal to 23% in the sleeping animal, an increase that allows the faster clearance of metabolic waste products and toxins.

Sleep to detox

It's likely that you feel refreshed after sleep because potentially neuro-toxic waste products of neural activity that build up in the central nervous system while you are awake are removed at an accelerated rate during sleep. When your brain is deprived of sleep the active process of your glymphatic system may not have the time it needs to give your brain the deep clean it requires to function well. Without this thorough clean, toxins can build up, preventing optimal brain function, impacting on your cognitive abilities, your behavior, and even your judgment during the day.

Disrupted sleep can harm or damage your cognitive function and may even contribute to the development of Alzheimer's disease. Mis-accumulation of cellular waste products is associated with almost all neurodegenerative diseases but the Alzheimer's–sleep link in particular has to do with the chemically sticky protein called amyloid.

It seems that sleeping doesn't just allow for deeper brain washing but also allows more efficient waste removal, with beta-amyloid being removed twice as fast in sleeping mice compared to awake mice. People living with Alzheimer's disease have abnormal clusters of the protein fragments called plaques in between nerve cells in their brain. Plaques form when pieces of beta-amyloid clump together. Small clumps may block signaling at synapses and may activate immune-system cells, triggering inflammation.

Neural cells are super sensitive to their environment, so it is vital that waste products are removed quickly. It is possible that lack of sleep plays a critical role in neurological conditions, such as Alzheimer's disease, by allowing byproducts to build up, leading to irreparable brain damage.

Nedergaard herself predicts: "You will probably develop damage if you don't get your sleep." She has also expressed concern for shift workers and questions the practice of medical staff waking brain-injury patients every ten minutes to check vital signs.

Of course, these studies were performed in mice so further research will be needed to confirm a similar waste-disposal system operates in the human brain. Scientists need to establish whether accelerated night-time "brain washing" occurs in humans.

Sleep cycles and stages

Your sleep-wake cycle is controlled at the molecular level by chemicals that act on neurons. Once you fall asleep you will pass through a number of different sleep stages.

Sleep pressure

The metabolic byproduct adenosine, which drives the pressure that you feel to sleep each evening, requires sleep in order to be cleared from your system. Adenosine plays a critical role in the sleep–wake cycle. As it rises throughout the day you feel a building pressure to sleep. During the afternoon its effect is countered by your circadian drive for arousal.

By late evening this circadian alerting system slackens off and the hormone melatonin is produced after dusk, calling you to sleep. While you sleep, adenosine gradually dissipates and the release of melatonin ceases in the early hours of morning.

A few hours before you wake your circadian rhythm increases its activity, transmitting an alerting signal throughout your brain and body.

The signal builds as the day progresses, reaching its peak in early afternoon.

You should feel wide awake throughout the morning due to the combination of a rising circadian alerting signal and low levels of adenosine. However, if you get insufficient sleep the adenosine won't have been fully cleared from your system, leaving you feeling groggy and tired instead of alert and refreshed.

Clock work

The timing of sleep is mainly controlled by your circadian clock, which is coordinated with the light–dark cycle over each twenty-four-hour period and so operates independently of the amount of sleep or wakefulness that you have experienced in the preceding period. The master conductor of your rhythm of life is a tiny structure called the superchiasmatic nucelus (SCN) within the hypothalamus[16] in your brain, which samples the light signals that travel from your eyes along the optic nerve at the point where they cross sides in your brain to travel toward your occipital lobe for visual processing. This information about light and darkness allows the SCN to synchronize your internal rhythms with your external environment.

Your SCN uses a circulating messenger called melatonin to communicate its repeating signal of night and day to your brain and your body. Soon after dusk, triggered by the SCN, melatonin is rapidly released into your bloodstream. Melatonin doesn't generate sleep or have any role in the sleep process, rather it is a messenger that runs through your bloodstream like a town crier yelling, "Oyez, oyez, night is nigh. It's time to sleep, it's time to sleep."

Over the course of the night, while you sleep, melatonin gradually dissipates from your system. The absence of melatonin informs your brain and body that it's time to end sleep and resume wakefulness. With dawn, the release of melatonin ceases and remains shut off completely during the hours of daylight until the cycle resumes again soon after dusk.

Sleep stages

Sleep has five stages, classified by whether rapid eye movement (REM) occurs or not: non-REM stages 1, 2, 3, 4, and REM. Your brain cycles through these five stages about five times each night, but each cycle is not identical because the ratio between non-REM and REM changes dramatically across the night. In the first half of the night most of your sleep is non-REM. During the second half of the night the amount of time spent in REM sleep, when you dream, increases. Your deepest sleep is experienced in non-REM sleep stages 3 and 4. Non-REM sleep is characterized by slow brainwaves interspersed with a burst of activity called spindles. In contrast, the electrical activity recorded during REM sleep is very similar to that of an awake brain.

Assessment: Sleep Log

Day 1 will be your first morning and the first day of your 100-Day Program.

Keep a Sleep Log for one week to help you to identify any patterns or personal habits that help or hinder your sleep quality. If you have a wrist activity tracker or sleep app on your phone or your watch you can use it to help you to complete this chart.

Complete in the morning	Day 1	Day 2	
Day (Mon, Tues, etc.)			
1. I went to bed last night at (time)			
2. I woke this morning at (time)			
3. I got out of bed at (time)			
4. I felt a) refreshed; b) somewhat refreshed; c) tired; d) groggy			
5. I had # hours, # minutes sleep, e.g., 06h 35m			
6. Last night I fell asleep after # minutes a) easily; b) with difficulty			
7. In the hour before bed I (list what you did, e.g., watched TV, took a bath, read a book, checked social media, online, worked, etc.)			
8. I woke during the night # times for # minutes			
9. I was woken by (list internal and external factors, such as a dream, thoughts, need to urinate, pain, dog, noise, too hot, too cold, breathing issues, coughing/ snoring, etc.)			

Day 3	Day 4	Day 5	Day 6	Day 7

Complete in the evening	Day 1	Day 2	
10. I exercised for # minutes today			
11. I exercised at (time)			
12. I consumed # caffeinated drinks			
13. I consumed caffeinated drinks at (time/s)			
14. I consumed # units of alcohol*			
15. I napped for # minutes at (time)			
16. I felt: a) alert; b) tired; c) drowsy Answer for morning, afternoon, and evening	M: A: E:	M: A: E:	
17. My mood was: awful (0) to great (5)			
18. Throughout the day I…(Answer yes/no)			
a) had trouble concentrating			
b) had difficulty shutting out distractions			
c) had trouble sustaining attention			
d) had trouble recalling information			
e) had trouble taking in new information			
f) felt irritable			
19. I took these medications			
20. I had my evening meal at (time)			
21. I consumed my last caffeinated drink at (time)			
22. I consumed my last alcoholic drink at (time)			

*750ml bottle of wine = 10 units, a single shot of spirits = 1 unit, a pint of strong beer = 3 units, and a pint of lower-strength beer = 2 units.

Use the information in this Sleep Log to answer Questions 1b, 2, 3, 4, 5b and 6 in Part Two of this chapter (Brain Health Goals: Sleep).

Refreshing

While you are awake your brain constantly acquires new information. Sleep refreshes your ability to learn and make new memories. Memory and learning are inextricably linked and different types of memory are processed in different parts of the brain. Declarative memory (memory for facts and events) involves the hippocampus, a part of the brain that temporarily accommodates the accumulation of new memories.

Day 3	Day 4	Day 5	Day 6	Day 7
M: A: E:	M: A: E:	M: A: E:	M: A: E:	M: A: E:

The synchronistic electrical activity of non-REM sleep allows distant regions of your brain to share information with each other promoting the strengthening of new learning and the consolidation of new memories.

During REM sleep this new information is integrated with existing information, experiences, and memories. This integration updates your internal model of the world, allowing you to solve problems, gain insight, and develop ideas. If you'd like more mornings where you wake with bright ideas and solutions, make sure you factor sufficient REM sleep into your sleep improvement plan.

Both non-REM and REM sleep are critical for brain health. In addition to getting the recommended number of hours' sleep each night, you also need to make sure that you are getting enough of both types of sleep.

Freeing up resources

There are limits to the capacity of the hippocampus, which sleep seems to solve.

Two groups of healthy adults with similar abilities were tasked with learning 100 face-name pairs. Afterward, one group took a ninety-minute nap while the other group stayed awake and engaged in mundane activities such as surfing the web or playing board games.

At 6 p.m., after the nap or activities, both groups were again put through their paces, learning a different batch of 100 face-name pairs. The "awake group" became progressively worse. In contrast the "nap group" actually improved, accruing a 20 percent learning advantage over their awake counterparts. Analysis of the electrical activity in their brains linked their learning replenishment to stage two, non-REM light sleep. The more spindles an individual had during their nap the more their ability to learn was restored.

More sleep spindles are also linked to greater restoration of the ability to learn after a full night's sleep. As we age, our brain's capacity to produce spindles diminishes to about 60 percent of the capacity we had as a young adult. Unfortunately, the fewer spindles we have when we sleep at night the poorer our learning capacity the following day.

A repeating loop of electrical current between the hippocampus and the cortex may reflect the transfer of newly acquired, fact-based information from the temporary repository of the hippocampus to a more permanent home in the cortex. This transfer frees up resources in the hippocampus, getting it ready to acquire new information on waking.

Making memories

The memory-making process has three sub-processes: encoding (also called acquisition), consolidation, and retrieval. During encoding, when you perceive something in your environment, a new fragile memory trace is formed. This labile memory trace is gradually stabilized through consolidation processes whereby the new knowledge is embedded within the brain ready for future retrieval.

Your awake brain is optimized for encoding and retrieval of information and your sleeping brain is optimized for memory consolidation. Sleep in the early part of the night is better than later in the night for retaining and saving memories, so make sure you factor this into your sleep improvement plan. The more deep, non-REM sleep you get the more facts you will be able to retain. When you recall facts immediately after you learn them you are activating your hippocampus. When you recall that same information after you get a good night's sleep, rich in deep non-REM sleep, you will activate your neocortex rather than your hippocampus. This is because during deep, non-REM sleep slow waves and sleep spindles transfer new information from the short-term memory repository of your hippocampus to a more stable permanent home in your neocortex.

In short, sleep before learning helps you to encode or acquire new information while sleep after learning helps you to consolidate memories.

The brain burns up a lot of energy and to be effective it also needs to be efficient. Every day your brain has to process a huge amount of information. Even though we have billions of neurons, synapses, and brain connections that are capable of processing masses of information, brain resources are not infinite.

It is not possible, nor does it make sense, for us to remember and consolidate every single piece of information or experience that we encounter, or retain every piece of information that we have ever remembered. In addition to consolidating memory, sleep may serve the purpose of discarding information that we don't need or information that we need to forget. A really interesting pattern of electrical activity that loops between the hippocampus and the frontal lobes 10 to 15 times during non-REM spindles could mean that the hippocampus checks in with the executive control unit in your frontal lobes. This is where information-filtering decisions about whether the information is important or irrelevant, to be remembered or to be discarded, are made.

No-Brainer: It's super important not to cut your sleep short otherwise you may impair your ability to learn new things.

Brain Drains: What Happens When Your Brain Is Deprived of Sleep?

When you get insufficient sleep your brain has to deal with both sleep deprivation and extended wakefulness, which are two different things. Sleep deprivation impacts on various aspects of cognitive functions including attention, learning, and memory.

The previous section outlined how sleep benefits the consolidation of memories after learning. Research on the impact of sleep loss on memory to date mainly focuses on hippocampal-dependent memory encoding, also known as acquisition, which happens before consolidation.

Sleep deprivation

When rodents are deprived of sleep, hippocampal neurogenesis, the growth of new neurons, is impaired. In addition, sleep loss reduces the production of proteins associated with neuroplasticity in the hippocampus.

In humans just one night of sleep deprivation impairs learning and encoding-related activity within the hippocampus. When people get a full night's sleep but are selectively deprived of non-REM, slow-wave sleep, encoding- and learning-related activity in the hippocampus is reduced. Sleep deprivation is also linked with impairments in larger brain networks.

Older adults show impairments in non-REM sleep and these impairments are magnified in people living with Alzheimer's disease. Greater impairment in learning and encoding in people with Alzheimer's disease is associated with lower levels of non-REM, slow-wave activity, and spindles.

I think most of us can attest to the fact that lack of sleep can make us irritable, anxious, emotionally unpredictable, and even aggressive. Without sleep you might also notice that it is harder to do things that require working memory, such as figuring out whether the girl on the till gave you the right amount of change or how to split the restaurant bill five ways. Sustained attention, which allows you to remain focused on a goal—such as reading a newspaper article to the end—is particularly vulnerable to sleep deprivation.

You might be less aware that sleep deprivation will make you more impulsive and more likely to take risks that you wouldn't consider with a full night's sleep. Sleep deprivation and low-quality sleep also impact on mood and, sadly, sleep loss also triggers changes in suicidal thoughts and suicide attempts. Your organs and systems also fall out of sync without sufficient sleep. In addition, there is a strong relationship between sleep loss and chronic stress, which is discussed in Chapter 4.

Without adequate sleep it becomes more difficult for your brain to receive and process information as your attention drifts and becomes unstable. Your neurons struggle to coordinate information, impacting on your ability to access previously learned information. Lapses of attention are nothing to be sneezed at as they can lead to accidents, injuries, and fatalities.

Given the negative impact of sleep deprivation on every aspect of your health, it is really important to identify factors that might disrupt your sleep so that you can address them in your action plan.

Assessment: Sleep Disruption

List each factor from Question 10 of your **Sleep Log** on a separate line under the column "I had trouble sleeping because." Then record the frequency at which each factor disrupted your sleep. If you did not experience a disruption this week check the "not this week" box.

However, if you feel that you did experience disruption "in the last month" then check that box instead and score as follows:

- Not during the past week = 0
- 1 or 2 times during the past week = 2
- 3 or more times during the past week = 3
- Less than once a week over the past month = 1

Sleep Disruptions	Based on your Sleep Log this week			In the past month	
I had trouble sleeping because:	Not this week	1 or 2 times	3 or more times	Less than once per week	Score
Total Score					

Total score = _____

What your score means
If total score is:

- 0 = No Sleep Disruption
- 1 to 9 inclusive = Low Sleep Disruption

- 10 to 18 inclusive = Moderate Sleep Disruption
- Greater than 18 = High Sleep Disruption

Transfer your score to Question 5a, Part Two of this chapter (Brain Health Goals: Sleep).

Sleep deprivation and dementia risk factors

Sleep deprivation can also play a role in the development of mid-life obesity and type 2 diabetes, both of which are associated with increased risk for Alzheimer's disease.

Obesity

Most of us are fully aware that we need to eat less and exercise more if we want to shift excess pounds and maintain a healthy weight. But did you know that insufficient sleep (less than seven or eight hours per night) can lead to weight gain and obesity? This seems counter-intuitive since you'd expect to burn more calories when awake and active than while sleeping. But sleeping is a metabolically active state, so staying up for twenty-four hours straight only burns an extra 147 calories when compared to the same period with eight hours sleep. However, the relationship between weight gain and sleep is more complex than the simple sum of calories burned. It involves multiple players, including two hormones (leptin and ghrelin) and your endocannabinoid system.

Hungry hormones

The hormone ghrelin triggers sensations of hunger while the hormone leptin signals feelings of fullness. Ever wondered why you feel starving when you burn the candle at both ends? It's because insufficient sleep decreases your levels of leptin and increases your levels of ghrelin, exposing you to the double whammy of an absent "stop eating" signal and an amplified "I'm still hungry" signal. As a consequence, the same amount of food that leaves you feeling satisfied the day after eight hours' sleep leaves you wanting more with half that amount of sleep.

Even with five to six hours sleep you are at risk of consuming 300 more calories a day than you would if you had adequate sleep. If you are regularly getting less than seven hours sleep per night it's easy to see how you might gain ten to fifteen pounds a year. On top of this, the less sleep you get the less energy you have and the more sedentary you become. When you are sleep deprived you not only eat more calories but in all probability you burn fewer, too. It's not unreasonable to draw a link between the sleep-loss epidemic and the obesity epidemic in industrial countries.

You've probably heard of marijuana-induced munchies, but did you know that your body naturally produces endocannabinoids, which are chemicals similar to the drug cannabis? Your endocannabinoid system plays a key role in your brain's appetite control and energy levels. When you are sleep deprived the level of endocannabinoids produced by your own body increase and stay in your system for longer than when you have had sufficient sleep.

In research studies, elevated levels of endocannabinoids coincide with people's reports of increased hunger and appetite. Sleep-deprived individuals consumed more in between meals and were more likely to consume unhealthy snacks than when they had sufficient sleep. The endocannabinoids appear to be driving pleasurable eating, also referred to as hedonic eating, which describes the drive to eat for pleasure in the absence of an energy deficit. With adequate sleep we have greater control, making it easier for us to resist junk food. In contrast, when we are sleep deprived our hedonic drive for specific foods increases and we are less able to resist them.

The sleep deprivation of the kind that many of us regularly engage in by choice not only leads us to eat more but also influences what we choose to eat, with cravings for sweets, salty foods, and heavy carbs increasing as our hours of nightly sleep decrease. In his book *Why We Sleep*, Matthew Walker describes an experiment that he conducted that offers further insight into the relationship between sleep loss and weight gain. His team found that lack of sleep seemed to silence brain activity in areas of the prefrontal cortex, which are involved in judgments and decision-making.

In parallel, lack of sleep amplifies brain activity in evolutionary older areas deep within your brain that drive desire and motivation. Sleep-deprived participants in his experiment consumed a staggering 600 more calories compared to when they had had adequate sleep. Thankfully, a full night's sleep restores the impulse control system necessary to reign in our more primal desire to eat to excess.

Unfortunately, poor sleep habits in childhood can set the stage for obesity in adulthood. Three-year-olds getting less than ten and a half hours of sleep per night have a 45 percent increased risk of being obese by age seven than those who get the recommended twelve hours of sleep per night.

Type 2 diabetes

In addition to increasing your risk of developing Alzheimer's disease, type 2 diabetes knocks a staggering ten years off your life. Blood sugar (glucose) is higher in individuals with type 2 diabetes than it is in healthy individuals. Over time, excessively high levels of glucose can have a devastating impact, leading to blindness, nerve damage, amputations, and kidney failure. Your pancreas produces a hormone called insulin, which controls glucose levels in your blood. After you eat, insulin is released, instructing your cells to open channels to absorb the influx of glucose from your meal to be used as energy. With type 2 diabetes the body becomes insulin-resistant and no longer uses insulin properly.

Rates of type 2 diabetes are higher in people who report regularly sleeping fewer than six hours a night, even when other risk factors for diabetes are taken into account. When healthy individuals have four hours sleep a night for just six nights they enter a pre-diabetic state of hyperglycemia. With less than a week of sleep deprivation they had become 40 percent less effective at absorbing glucose and were they to go to their doctor they would be classified as pre-diabetic.

It seems that the cells of sleep-deprived individuals become unresponsive to the instruction from insulin to open their channels. Rather than absorbing glucose their cells repel insulin, leading to dangerously high blood sugar levels. This pre-diabetic state can even occur with less-severe sleep debt and as a consequence chronic sleep deprivation is now considered a serious risk factor for developing type 2 diabetes, which in turn increases risk for developing dementia.

> **No-Brainer**: Invest in sleep to protect your health, preserve memory, and minimize accidents.

Summary

- When it comes to sleep and brain health, both quantity and quality matter:
  - Get the recommended number of hours sleep every night;
  - Your brain needs both non-REM and REM sleep, so get your sleep at the right time, preferably beginning at some point between 8 p.m. and midnight.
- New information is strengthened and new memories consolidated during non-REM sleep.
- New information is integrated with existing information, experiences, and memories during REM sleep, allowing you to solve problems, gain insight, and develop ideas.
- As we get older we don't need less sleep but we may experience a decline in the quantity, quality, and efficiency of our sleep.
- The only thing that can relieve sleep pressure and rid your system of adenosine is sleep.
- Work with light to optimize sleep.
- Sleep is critical for clearing the brain of toxins.
- Sleep is critical for learning, memory, and attention.
- Sleep deprivation interferes with neuroplasticity, impairs various cognitive functions, and leads to weight gain.
- Just one week of sleep deprivation can send you into a pre-diabetic state.

Brain Changers: What You Can Do

In this section you will find down-to-earth suggestions that will help you to develop your sleep improvement goals and action plan.

Sleep is fundamental to brain health—reframe it as an elixir for your brain. Sleep is an investment in your future that costs you nothing but time spent sleeping soundly in your bed each night.

TEN PRACTICAL TIPS TO CHERISH SLEEP

1. Go to bed and get up at the same time each day.
2. Unwind and create a calming bedtime ritual.
3. Manage light exposure.
4. Create a sleep haven.
5. Get physically active during the day.
6. Quit smoking.
7. Avoid caffeine in the evenings.
8. Avoid alcohol close to bedtime.
9. Manage conditions or medications that impact on sleep quality.
10. Manage stress.

1. Go to bed and get up at the same time each day

The assessments in this chapter will help you to devise a personal sleep schedule that takes account of your age, your work commitments, and any relevant lifestyle factors. Stick to your schedule— that means going to bed and getting up at the same time every day regardless of whether it is the weekend or your day off. Sleep is not a luxury, it is absolutely essential for physical, mental, and brain health. Make sure that you are getting the recommended amount of sleep every night at the very least.

Both non-REM and REM sleep are critical for brain health. In addition to getting the recommended number of hours sleep each night for your age you also need to make sure that you are getting enough of both types of sleep. Remember, your brain gets proportionately more non-REM in the earlier part of the night and proportionately more REM in the early hours of the morning.

So if you are getting fewer than the recommended hours of sleep because you regularly go to bed after midnight, you may be depriving your brain of the time to carry out the important activities of non-REM sleep. Conversely, if you regularly cut short your sleep by getting up ultra early you may be depriving your brain of a large proportion of the time needed to carry out the activities of REM sleep.

2. Unwind and create a calming bedtime ritual

Create a calming, relaxing bedtime ritual that doesn't include light-emitting devices—so if reading helps you to relax, read printed books or listen to audio books. I've recently discovered podcasts and find them very effective for winding down—to the extent that the next day I need to rewind the podcast back to the point where I fell asleep!

A warm bath can be deeply relaxing as the rise and fall in body temperature induces drowsiness. Some people may find that bathing before bedtime wakes them up, though; it's very individual. Experiment until you find a ritual that works for you.

Meditation or mindfulness can be calming and can also guard against reliving the past or worrying about the future. Meditation isn't everyone's cup of tea but simply being present-minded, focusing on what you are doing while you are doing it, in the thirty minutes before bed, can be very effective.

Consider making a happiness journal as part of your night-time ritual. Simply get a notebook or journal and each evening as part of your pre-bedtime ritual write down one thing that made you happy that day—it can be as simple as seeing a flower come into bloom or hearing a baby gurgle. I find that when I do this it helps to orient my day toward positivity, as I look for positive things throughout the day for my evening entry. Experiment until you find a routine that works for you. You can read more about the brain-health benefits of positivity in Chapter 8.

3. Manage light exposure

Make sure your bedroom is as dark as possible at night, as this will help you to sleep. Artificial blue light is emitted from digital devices and from LED lighting. Avoid blue-light exposure for an hour before sleep and avoid it altogether in the bedroom. If you wake in the night don't be tempted to reach for your phone or laptop because the device's blue light will wake your brain and make it difficult to get back to sleep. Make your bedroom a technology-free zone. Get yourself a traditional clock to check the time and to use as an alarm. This will prevent you falling down the rabbit hole of checking the time on your phone, which not only exposes you to blue light but also increases the risk of clicking on email or social media notifications.

Invest in a dimmer switch for your bedroom and bathroom so that you can lower the lights before you retire to bed. Consider altering your bedroom routine so that brushing your teeth under bright lights in the bathroom is not the very last thing that you do before you go to bed. Switch up the order of your night-time habits a little, maybe brush your teeth at the start of your wind-down routine rather than at the end of it. Make sure you have a safe route to the bathroom should you wake during the night, but if possible avoid switching on ultra-bright lights. Low-level night-lights can guide the way. A bedside torch and dimmer switches en route can all help.

Make sure that you get exposure to natural light for at least thirty minutes every day, you can combine this with other brain-health activities such as taking physical exercise or socializing with friends. If you can, try to get exposure to morning sunlight, open the shutters or curtains as soon as possible after waking. If you live in a part of the world where the mornings are dark, expose yourself to bright light as soon as you wake up (bright, not blue).

In later life melatonin release reaches its peak earlier in the evening, nudging you toward an earlier bedtime. You may struggle to stay awake in the evening, but if you inadvertently nod off mid-evening it counts as a nap, which unfortunately dilutes sleep pressure to the extent that you may struggle to get to sleep when you eventually go to bed in the evening. In addition, as you get older your circadian clock also tends to wake you up earlier in the morning. If you continually refuse to take account of the changing rhythms and pressures of your body you will push yourself further and further into sleep debt. You can respond to the pressure to sleep earlier or, alternatively, sleep researcher Matthew Walker suggests tailoring your light exposure to gain greater control over age-related changes in your circadian rhythm by getting more exposure to natural light in the afternoons, so that you push out the time at which melatonin is released.

4. Create a sleep haven

Take stock of your bedroom. Use all of your senses to really examine everything in your room and ask yourself the following questions:

- Are the colors on your walls calming and conducive to sleep?
- How effective are your curtains or shutters at blocking light?
- Is your room cluttered?
- Does everything that you have in your bedroom need to be there or could it be stored somewhere else in the house or dumped?
- How tidy is your bedroom?
- How dusty is your bedroom?
- When was the last time you changed your pillows or your mattress?
- How comfortable are your bedclothes?
- Are there smells in your room that might hinder your sleep?
- Are there noises that could intrude on your sleep?
- How much technology is there in your bedroom?
- Are there items in your bedroom that could lead to stress, worry, or anxiety?
- How comfortable is the temperature of your bedroom?

Answering these questions will help you to identify some physical barriers to sleep. Some will be easy to fix, while others may take time and cost money. Add them to your action plan in the next section and prioritize them in the context of the importance of sleep.

Weigh up the cost of revamping your bedroom against the value that sleep has for your health. If your living arrangements permit, try to make your bedroom a haven for sleep, avoid dual-purpose use such as home office or TV watching. Many teen and kids' bedrooms are dual-purpose—filled with toys and consoles and often desks for study. If at all possible, try to avoid this, but if space limitations make this unavoidable, find ways to transform the room from day use to sleep haven by shutting down and removing devices and tidying toys and study or work materials away. There are lots of ingenious storage solutions that will allow you to do this.

5. Get physically active during the day

Physical activity is great for brain health and can also work wonders in terms of improving your sleep pattern and sleep quality, provided you don't exercise within two to three hours of your bespoke bedtime. You can read more about the brain-health benefits of physical activity in Chapter 7, where you will also find more detailed practical tips about how to get physically active.

6. Quit smoking

Nicotine is a stimulant. If your plan is to cut down on the number of cigarettes that you smoke gradually rather than go cold turkey, avoid nicotine, including patches and gum, for at least an hour before bedtime. You will find more suggestions and detailed information on the impact of smoking on brain health in Chapter 6.

7. Avoid caffeine in the evenings

Caffeine is a psychoactive stimulant. When you consume drinks containing caffeine you feel stimulated and alert because the caffeine dampens the effect of the sleep-pressure chemical adenosine. Caffeine doesn't get rid of adenosine from your system, though, nor does it magically pay off your sleep debt. Caffeine just blocks the sleepiness signal, tricking you into feeling alert. The sleep pressure is still there, you still need to sleep and the sleep debt continues to build.

Caffeine persists in your system for quite some time after consumption — depending on the individual it can take five to seven hours to clear just half of it. As you get older the time it takes your brain and body to process and remove caffeine from your system increases. Try not to consume caffeine within four to five hours of bedtime and remember various products, including decaffeinated coffee, contain caffeine.

8. Avoid alcohol close to bedtime

Don't be fooled by the fact that alcohol initially makes you sleepy; it can disrupt sleep later in the night. After a few hours alcohol acts as a stimulant that interferes with the quality of your sleep. Ditch the nightcap and avoid drinking alcohol within three hours of bedtime. Try to limit consumption to two units or less and avoid binge-drinking large quantities of alcohol.

9. Manage conditions or medications that impact on sleep quality

If you take medications and experience difficulty falling asleep, staying asleep, daytime drowsiness, or other disruptions in your sleep patterns, it might be worth a visit to your doctor to see whether the medication is the culprit.

Some heart, blood-pressure, and asthma medications can interfere with sleep, as can over-the-counter cold, flu, and headache tablets. The chemicals in these medications don't always affect everyone in the same way.

Don't stop prescribed medications of your own accord, always consult with your doctor to find alternative treatments that don't impact on your sleep.

If you are kept awake by the symptoms of a chronic condition it may well be worth speaking to a health professional to learn about ways to improve your sleep quality.

10. Manage stress

Poorly managed chronic stress can interfere with sleep. If stresses and worries tend to keep you awake at night or wake you during the night, set aside time earlier in the day to focus on addressing whatever it is that is worrying or stressing you.

Alternatively, you can write down your worries in a journal. The act of putting them onto the page can get them out of your head. If the worries intrude on your bedtime ritual or wake you during the night, acknowledge them and make it explicit to yourself that you will deal with them at a specified time the next day. You can read more about how stress impacts brain health in the next chapter, where you will also find more detailed practical tips to manage stress.

SLEEP—PART TWO

Goals—Action Plan—Personal Profile

Set your goals, devise your action plan, and create your personal profile for Sleep.

Brain Health Goals: Sleep

Answering the following questions will help you to set sleep-improvement goals to boost your brain health. (You can find a completed sample in the back of the book.)

Q1. Sleep duration

The National Sleep Foundation recommends 7–9 hours sleep for adults aged 18 to 64 and 7–8 hours sleep for adults aged over 65 each night. Given the variability in sleep duration needs, you might find that slightly more and/or slightly less sleep is appropriate for you. However, you should not get less than 5 hours or more than 9 hours each night. Adults under 65 should not get less than 6 hours sleep each night. Adults aged 26–64 should get no more than 10 hours and no more than 11 hours if they are between the ages of 18 and 25.

a) Base your answer on the recommendations above

How many hours sleep do you need each night to optimize your
     health?____

I am getting
too little sleep ☐   too much sleep ☐   the right amount of sleep ☐

b) Base your answer on the information in your *Assessment: Sleep Log*

On average* how many hours' sleep do you get each night?_____

*To calculate your average, convert your sleep for each night to minutes, add them together, then divide your answer by seven and convert back to hours and minutes.

How did this compare to your estimate at the start of the chapter?

Sleep Goal No. 1

a) I want to gain _____ hours or lose _____ hours sleep each night.

b) No action required: I am getting the recommended number of hours' sleep ☐

Q2. Sleep schedule

Base your answer on the information in your *Assessment: Sleep Log*

I have no regular pattern, I go to bed at different times most nights ☐

I have no regular pattern, I get out of bed at different times most mornings ☐

I go to bed at the same time most days: Yes ☐ No ☐

I usually go to bed at _____ on weekdays/workdays

I usually go to bed at _____ on weekends/days off

I get up at the same time most days: Yes ☐ No ☐

I usually get out of bed at _____ on weekdays/workdays

I usually get out of bed at _____ on weekends/days off

I get _____ hours' sleep before midnight most nights

The optimal window of opportunity for starting sleep is between 8 p.m. and midnight. A good rule of thumb is to count backward from the time you need to/would like to/usually wake at.

In order to get sufficient non-REM and REM sleep:

My optimum time to go to sleep is _____

My optimum time to wake is _____

Experiment to find your personal optimal sleep pattern, taking into account your age, your work, your personal preferences and any other time-critical responsibilities.

Sleep Goal No. 2

I want to work on going to bed at the same time each night:
Yes ☐ No ☐

I want to work on getting up at the same time each morning:
Yes ☐ No ☐

No action required: I have a regular sleep pattern ☐

Q3. Difficulty getting to sleep

Base your answer on the information in your *Assessment: Sleep Log*

I usually have difficulty getting to sleep: Yes ☐ No ☐

This week it took me more than thirty minutes to get to sleep:
3 or more times ☐ 1 or 2 times ☐ not during the past week ☐

Sleep Goal No. 3

I want to determine the factors that are interfering with my ability to get to sleep ☐

No action required: I fall asleep easily each night ☐

Q4. Sleep quality

Base your answer on the information in your *Assessment: Sleep Log*

How would you rate the quality of your sleep overall over the past week?

Excellent ☐ Very good ☐ Fairly good ☐
Fairly poor ☐ Very poor ☐

Most days on getting out of bed I felt:

Refreshed ☐ Fairly refreshed ☐ Tired ☐ Groggy ☐

Sleep Goal No. 4

I want to determine the factors that are interfering with the quality of my sleep ☐

No action required: I am happy with the quality of my sleep ☐

Q5. Sleep disruption and impact

a) My *Assessment: Sleep Disruption* score is:

None ☐   Low ☐   Moderate ☐   High ☐

Sleep Goal No. 5

I want to identify and address the factors that regularly disrupt my sleep ☐

No action required: I sleep through the night ☐

No action required: I wake briefly (e.g., for the bathroom) but get back to sleep easily ☐

b) Based on the information in my *Assessment: Sleep Log*, my sleep habits may be interfering with my (tick all that apply):

Alertness ☐   Mood ☐   Concentration ☐   Attention ☐
Memory ☐   Irritability ☐

Not interfering ☐

Q6. Sleep barriers

Base your answers on the information your *Assessment: Sleep Log* and your usual habits

a) Thinking about your usual caffeine consumption:

I don't drink coffee   (skip to section 6b)

I can function optimally without caffeine before lunch:
Yes ☐   No ☐

I may be self-medicating with caffeine to counteract sleep debt:
Yes ☐   No ☐

My caffeine consumption is ___ cups per day, starting at ___ ending at ___

Sleep Goal No. 6a

I want to reduce the amount of caffeine I consume each day:
Yes ☐   No ☐

I want to pull back the time I have my last cup of coffee to
___ o'clock each day

No action required: my caffeine consumption does not impact on
my sleep Yes ☐   No ☐

---

b) Thinking about your usual bedtime:

I frequently find that I am wide awake at bedtime: Yes ☐   No ☐

I usually feel sleepy at bedtime: Yes ☐   No ☐

I read in bed on a light-emitting device: Yes ☐   No ☐

I regularly watch TV or stream content on a device in bed:
Yes ☐   No ☐

I have a regular wind-down routine before bedtime: Yes ☐   No ☐

Sleep Goal No. 6b

I want to alter my use of light-emitting devices at bedtime:
Yes ☐   No ☐

I want to develop a wind-down routine before bedtime:
Yes ☐   No ☐

No action required: my wind-down routine excludes light-emitting
devices ☐

Completing the table below using the information from your Sleep Goals will help you to characterize your current healthy habits and prioritize any sleep habits that need fixing. Tick the box that applies then enter any items that need fixing into the Brain Health Action Plan on the next page.

	Healthy	Needs fixing	Priority*
Number of hours' sleep per night			
Regular sleep schedule			
Time to bed—I get sufficient non-REM			
Time to rise—I get sufficient REM			
Daily physical exercise			
Daily exposure to light			
Nightly wind-down routine			
Use of light-emitting devices			
Bedroom environment			
Caffeine consumption			
Nicotine consumption			
Alcohol consumption			
Meal time—eating at night			
Other			

* High, medium, or low

Brain Health Action Plan: Sleep

Enter your sleep habits that "need fixing" into the "Brain Health Action" column in the table opposite. Indicate whether the action is attainable with relative ease in the short term (quick fix) or will require more time and effort to achieve (long term). The ten tips that you have just read should help you to break each action into practical steps. Prioritize the actions in the order you would like to work on them (1 = tackle first).

Brain Health Action	Order	Steps	Quick fix	Long term

Personal Profile: Sleep

Using your scores in the **Brain Health Goals: Sleep** section as a guide, complete this table. Indicate whether your scores are healthy, borderline, or unhealthy. From that you can determine whether your current pattern of behavior is a brain-healthy asset or a risk that could compromise your brain health and make you vulnerable to dementia in later life. Finally, indicate the aspects that you would like to fix, improve, or maintain and prioritize them for inclusion in your bespoke Brain Health Plan in Chapter 9. *You will find a completed sample in the back of the book.*

Aspect	Healthy	Borderline	Unhealthy	Asset	Risk	Maintain	Improve	Fix	Priority
Duration									
Schedule									
Quality									
Disruption									
Barriers									
Total									

100 Days to a Younger Brain

PROGRAM DAYS 1–7: CHERISHING SLEEP

You now have a clear understanding of your current sleep patterns, your personal goals, and the actions that you need to take to transform your sleep habit to benefit your brain health. You will combine your sleep profile with the other profiles that you will create as you complete this program to build your overall Brain Health Profile in Chapter 9. You will also select at least one of your sleep actions to add to your overall Brain Health Plan.

100-DAY DIARY

You can record the steps that you are taking toward your program goals in the 100-Day Diary at the back of the book, for example:

- I bought an old-school alarm clock.
- I had a bath before bed.

- I left my phone to charge downstairs overnight rather than beside my bed.
- I decluttered my bedroom.

You can also celebrate your healthy habits by recording them in your 100-Day Diary.

4
Manage Stress

"The greatest weapon against stress is our ability to choose one thought over another."
William James

STRESS—PART ONE

A little bit of stress can go a long way, motivating you to attain your goals and meet daily challenges. In fact, well-managed stress will support you through challenge and change, making you more resilient and better equipped for whatever life throws at you. *Stress in the short term can enhance your memory function, but poorly managed chronic stress and persistently high levels of stress hormones can actually inhibit learning and impair memory function, impacting negatively on the size, structure, and function of your brain.*

Managing and monitoring the stressors in your life and your response to them is critical if you want to keep your brain healthy. The stress response, also commonly known as the "fight or flight" response, evolved to allow humans and other mammals to fight off a threat or turn the other way and run like hell from it. Physical stressors such as illness, injury, and pain can lead to the release of stress hormones, but you can also experience psychological stress when you perceive that the demands placed on you exceed your ability to cope.

In this chapter you will find ten practical tips to help you manage stress. Keeping the Life Balance Log and Stress Log and completing the other assessments in this chapter will give you insight into how you perceive stress, as well as a snapshot of your current stress levels, which will help you to identify your stress sweet spot, which will in turn benefit your brain health. You will use this information to create your personal stress profile, set goals, and devise a stress action plan in Part Two of this chapter.

First, let's determine what stress is, what happens in your brain in response to stress, and the impact that poorly managed chronic stress can have on brain health.

Quick Question: Average Stress

In the last month, my average stress level across the whole month was _____

Where 1 = completely calm all of the time and 10 = totally stressed all of the time.

Brain Gains: What Is Stress?

The word stress is frequently used interchangeably in conversation to mean the thing that stresses you, the physiological changes that occur in your body, as well as the psychological and neurobiological aspects of the phenomenon. In a sense stress is all of these things, but to avoid confusion it is helpful to distinguish specific aspects.

The body's stress response evolved to allow you to respond to a threat in a way that gives you the best chance of survival and also keeps you healthy while you respond to that threat.

So let's call the "threat," the thing that stresses you, the **_stressor_**.

A stressor kicks off a sequence of coordinated neurophysiological events in your brain and body. These events allow you to fight or take flight and then return your body to the status quo (homeostasis), which is the optimum condition that has been disturbed by the stressor.

Let's call this neurophysiological response the **_stress response_**.

In the early part of the twentieth century, stress was originally described in the context of acute physical crisis, such as illness or injury. However, over time researchers came to understand that the stress response could also be activated by psychological states such as the loss of social support, perceived loss of control, and the absence of predictability in our lives. **Psychological stress** refers to the extent to which a person perceives that their demands exceed their ability to cope.

Roller blades and roller coasters

The body's neurophysiological stress response will kick in whether the perceived threat is real or imagined, and will do so in response to different stressors for different people. It is very individual; some people seek out risky situations while others avoid them. You might ride roller coasters while I won't even ride rollerblades. Having said that, while there are dramatic differences from one individual to the next about whether an event or an internal state is stressful, some things, such as a life-threatening injury, a major burn or an altercation with a violent attacker, will reliably activate the stress response.

The stress response helps you maintain your health while you respond to the stressor. However, experiencing severe or prolonged stress can negatively impact on your health and be particularly harmful to your central nervous system, affecting your behavior and your brain function, including your ability to learn and remember. Chronic stress can also lead to or increase your risk of mental and physical illness and disease.

We tend to think of stress as a bad thing, but having an optimal amount of stress in your life is important as it motivates you to attain your goals, and allows you to adapt to your changing environment and meet daily challenges. The total absence of stress is associated with boredom and disengagement, neither of which is good for your brain health or indeed your mental health.

The acute neurophysiological response to stress protects your body and your brain and helps reestablish or maintain your body's stable state. This counteracts influences that might lead to deviation from the optimal state at which it evolved to function best.

The stress response depends on the type of stressor, its intensity, and how long it lasts. Broadly speaking, the effects of stress follow what is known as an inverted U-shaped dose-response curve that is a function of stressor severity. This just means that the effects of mild to moderate stress (visualized in the arc or optimal zone of the upside-down U) are beneficial. While the complete absence of stress and severe and/or prolonged stress (visualized on the left and right sides of the inverted-U respectively) have harmful effects on your brain.

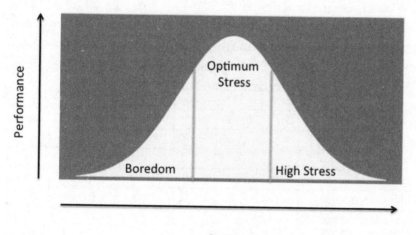

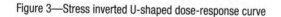

Figure 3—Stress inverted U-shaped dose-response curve

Under stimulation

Images of the thousands of Romanian orphans shocked the world when they were first exposed in 1989. Even if their physical needs were met, their emotional needs were ignored and they were deprived of stimulation, including play and emotional support. These children are a testament to the impact of an under-stimulatory environment. The EEGs (measures of electrical activity in the brain) of children who had been in the orphanages since birth showed reduced neural activity, the children also had other signs of an underdeveloped brain and their language was severely delayed. There are other less extreme examples of under-stimulation, such as those that can occur with unemployment and social isolation.

Severe and chronic stress can impact on physical health, mental health, and brain health, leading to compromised immunity, anxiety, impaired memory, and more.

Assessment: Life Balance Log

Keep a **Life Balance Log** for one week, starting on Day 8 of your *100 Days to a Younger Brain*. Use the table below to note the amount of time you spend each day doing the activities listed. You don't have to be exact. Do try to complete this table each day to get an accurate sense of the proportion of your day spent in each activity. If you spend a significant portion of your time doing something that is not listed, note the amount of time and list the activity beside "Other." *You will find a completed sample in the back of the book.*

Activity	Day 1	Day 2	Day 3	Day 4	Day 5	Day 6	Day 7
Day (Mon, Tues, etc.)							
Work							
Housework*							
Time with family							
Time when work intruded on personal life							
Time when personal life intruded on work life							
Exercise							
Hobbies/interests							
Indoors							
Outdoors							
Smiling/laughing							
Sleeping							
Other _____							

*Include house-related chores such as shopping, cleaning, cooking, gardening, etc.

Use the information you record in this Life Balance Log to answer Question 4 in Part Two (Brain Health Goals: Stress).

Assessment: Stress Log

On Days 8–14, keep a log of any stress that you experience. If you don't experience any stress, leave the log blank. If you have more than one stress experience in any day, note down each one. This will help you to identify patterns. *You will find a completed sample in the back of the book.*

Duration: The total time from when you began feeling stressed to when you returned to feeling calm.

Stressor: The thing, thought, person, situation, event, etc., that led to your feelings of stress.

Location: Where you were, e.g., at work, home, supermarket, highway.

Activity: What you were doing at the time, e.g., dealing with a customer, solving a problem, arguing, parenting, thinking, trying to sleep.

Level: The level your stress reached at its peak: 1 = mild, 2 = moderate, 3 = strong, 4 = severe.

Regular: Indicate the number of times you have felt stressed by this particular stressor in the past month.

Coping strategy: Indicate any strategy you used to cope with the experience.

Day	Time	Duration	Stressor	Location	Activity	Level	Regular	Coping strategy

Use the information in this Stress Log to answer Question 3 in Part Two of this Chapter (Brain Health Goals: Stress).

From comfort zone to optimal zone

In the context of brain health the aim is not to eliminate stress but to identify your own individual stress sweet spot, where stress is optimal for you, where you subjectively experience stimulation, arousal, alertness, engagement, and even fun. You will most likely find this at the boundaries of safety and risk, control and freedom, excitement and fear, where learning, growth, achievement, and change occur and where fun and vitality can reside. It is usually transient and is different for everyone.

Challenge, novelty, and learning are vital for brain health. Your personal stress sweet spot resides where you feel safe enough to step outside your comfort zone to challenge yourself and enjoy new experiences, thereby enriching not just your life but also your brain through learning. By operating within this optimal zone you give your brain the opportunity to adapt in an ever-changing world, building resilience by remodeling its own neural architecture.

What happens when my stress response is activated?

Your amazing brain doesn't just adapt to the social, psychological, and physical stressors that challenge you, it also determines what is threatening, accumulates pertinent memories and regulates your physiological and behavioral responses. There are two key systems involved in the stress response: the fast-acting autonomic nervous system[17] and the slower hypothalamic-pituitary-adrenal (HPA) axis. The amygdala, the hippocampus, and the prefrontal cortex are also of particular interest in terms of the impact of stress on brain health.

As adrenaline[18] circulates through your body it triggers physiological changes that happen so quickly you aren't consciously aware of them. Your heart beats faster than normal, pumping blood to your muscles. Your sweat glands contract, squeezing sweat droplets onto your skin. Your breathing speeds up so you can take in as much oxygen as possible, and your brain receives extra oxygen, increasing alertness. Your sight, hearing, and other senses become sharper. Energy-providing glucose (blood sugar) is released into your bloodstream.

The long and the short of the stress response

Your amygdala and your hypothalamus set all of this in motion before your visual system has had a chance to fully process what is happening. Sensory information travels to your amygdala via two separate routes: a short pathway and a long pathway.

The sensory information is first routed to your amygdala via your thalamus,[19] leading to your first, fast, startled reaction (short route).

Sensory information is also sent from your thalamus to your cortex for processing in areas including your prefrontal cortex and then on to your amygdala (long route).

Your cortex evaluates the information and assigns meaning and determines whether the situation is threatening or not, then your amygdala is informed and produces an appropriate response.

The long route brings your awareness to the actuality of the situation, allowing you to establish whether you are in danger or you have in fact been startled by a harmless noise.

The changes happen so quickly that you aren't consciously aware of them, but they will save your life, getting you to jump back out of the way of a speeding oncoming car without having to think about it.

After the threat has passed, your parasympathetic system[20] takes over and brings your body back to a balanced state.

Cortisol

Within fifteen to twenty minutes of a stressful event, cortisol is released. Cortisol has become known as the stress hormone, but almost every cell in your body carries receptors for cortisol, so it can have lots of different actions, depending on the type of cell that it is acting on. In the context of the stress response, the stressor activates your HPA axis.

Cortisol mobilizes energy to respond to the demands of your behavioral response to the stressor by either activating or suppressing different processes in your body. An adequate and steady supply of blood sugar will allow you to cope with a prolonged stressor. Cortisol may also suppress processes not essential for survival in the moment, such as immunity, digestion, and growth.

The release of cortisol is regulated by what is known as a negative feedback mechanism, which means that as cortisol levels rise they block the release of hormones, ultimately leading to a drop in cortisol levels.

Cortisol gets a terribly bad rap really, because everyone associates it with the negative aspects of chronic stress, but you need a steady stream of cortisol in your blood for lots of your basic functions. For example, it is secreted into your blood in a predictable twenty-four-hour rhythm. Your natural body clock, your circadian rhythm, reaches a peak in cortisol in the early morning, producing a wake-up signal, getting you out of bed, and turning on appetite and physical activity. Then your cortisol levels decline slowly over the course of the day, reaching a maximum low around bedtime. It rises again in the early night-time hours, slowly preparing for the morning to ensure that you have lots of energy to face the new day.

Memory

The release of the stress hormones cortisol and adrenaline in an acute response enhance muscular activity so that you have the strength to fight or the speed to flee. Stress hormones also flow to your hippocampus to help you remember those notable moments and make you aware of the potential danger, and to support your survival in the future.

Memory is enhanced so that you remember the event and are reminded not to go down that dark alley, or so that you can recall how you managed to overcome or escape your attacker. Once the threat has passed the stress response restores physiological balance, cortisol levels return to baseline, and your nervous system shifts you from fight or flight to rest-and-digest mode. Chronic stress can disrupt this natural rhythm, interfering with circadian rhythms and sleep, which, as you know from reading Chapter 3, is vital for brain health.

No-Brainer: Strive for the optimum amount of stress in your life to allow you to enjoy new experiences, thereby enriching your brain and your life.

Brain Drains: What Happens to Your Brain When Stress Becomes Chronic?

From the early days of stress research it has been appreciated that prolonged stress increases the likelihood that you will be sick. A stressor that continues for extended periods can repeatedly elevate neurophysiological stress responses or fail to shut them off when they are not needed. When this occurs, the same physiological mechanisms that are helpful in an acute situation can upset your body's biochemical balance, accelerating disease and affecting your brain function.

Chronic stress

Over long periods of time, if stress hormones continue to be released, the consequences can be negative. Memory is impaired, immune function remains suppressed and excess energy is stored as fat. If left unchecked this can lead to hardening of the arteries, abdominal obesity, and high blood pressure, all of which in turn increase your risk of developing dementia and lead to loss of brain volume and impaired ability to learn and remember.

Our bodies are usually very efficient and, thanks to the negative feedback mechanism, cortisol levels are kept under control. However, when cortisol levels are too high for too long it seems this feedback mechanism gets a little screwed up. Cortisol production may go through the roof or your body may not make enough of it. Or you may make a ton of it at night when you are trying to sleep and nothing in the morning when you need it to get out of bed. Ugh. Essentially your cortisol levels become out of sync with your needs.

Assessment: Perceived Stress

This assessment asks you about your feelings and thoughts during the last month to establish how you perceive stress. In each case, indicate by entering the score that reflects how often you felt or thought a certain way. While the questions might seem similar they are different, so treat each one as a separate question. Answer fairly quickly. Don't try to count up the number of times you felt a particular way in the last month, instead tick the answer that is the best estimate.

In the past month...	Never 0	Almost never 1	Some-times 2	Fairly often 3	Very often 4
1. How often have you been upset because of something that happened unexpectedly?					
2. How often have you felt that you were unable to control the important things in your life?					
3. How often have you felt nervous and "stressed"?					
4. How often have you felt confident about your ability to handle your personal problems?					
5. How often have you felt that things were going your way?					
6. How often have you found that you could not cope with all the things that you had to do?					
7. How often have you been able to control irritations in your life?					
8. How often have you felt that you were on top of things?					
9. How often have you been angered because of things that were outside of your control?					
10. How often have you felt difficulties were piling up so high that you could not overcome them?					

To calculate your score:

First, reverse your scores for Questions 4, 5, 7, and 8.

On these 4 questions, change the scores as follows:

Never = 4, Almost never = 3, Sometimes = 2, Fairly often = 1,

Very often = 0.

Now add up your scores for each item to get a total.

My total score is _____

What your score means

Individual scores on the scale can range from 0–40, with higher scores indicating higher levels of perceived stress.

Scores ranging from 0–13 are considered low stress.

Scores ranging from 14–26 are considered moderate stress.

Scores ranging from 27–40 are considered high perceived stress.

Note: If you are concerned about your stress levels, irrespective of how you score on the scales in this chapter, it might be a good idea to speak with your doctor.

Transfer your score to Question 2b, Part Two of this chapter (Brain Health Goals: Stress)

Psychological stress

How you perceive stress is important. Psychological stress is a risk factor for age-related decline in cognitive function. More than 5.4 million adults aged over seventy living in the United States have cognitive impairment without dementia. Tackling modifiable risk factors such as psychological stress can minimize the risk of cognitive impairment and indeed dementia in later life. Psychological stress is an important risk factor because it is also related to a number of health outcomes that, in turn, increase risk of cognitive decline and dementia.

When you appraise a situation or event as stressful you allocate cognitive resources to coping. This results in a lower cognitive performance than during non-stressful times. If you are preoccupied with a stressor and find yourself either replaying a past stressful encounter over and over or worrying about some event that might happen at some point in the future, it impacts on your cognitive functioning in the here and now. This is because your rumination is consuming your limited attention and eating into resources needed for ongoing information processing.

In these circumstances, short-term stress impacts on your cognitive functioning by reducing your ability to pay attention, to keep track of what you are doing or saying or to remember steps in a task at hand. This kind of stress is associated with short-term increases in inflammation and negative mood, both of which are associated with fatigue, which might explain reductions in your capacity to pay attention.

Chronic stress in the long term is consistently associated with poorer cognitive performance, increased incidence of dementia and accelerated cognitive decline compared to the rate of decline observed in less-stressed peers. Chronic stress increases biological wear and tear, hormones get messed up, inflammation is increased, and the neural structure that underlies cognitive function undergoes stress-induced changes.

What has stress got to do with memory?

You don't need me to tell you that emotion and memory are very closely linked. You know that they are from your own experience. When you meet a bunch of new people at a party, who will you remember from the evening? You will, of course, remember the one who made you laugh or the one who made you feel embarrassed or the one you argued with. Over time your strongest, most persistent memories will have some sort of emotional salience for you, and that personal meaning, that significance, can run the range of emotions from pleasure to pain and from fun to fear.

In addition to preparing you for the acute consequences of a threat and the return to homeostasis, stress also serves the important function of bringing about long-term adaptive responses. Enhanced memory for emotionally significant experiences and stressful events is highly adaptive and allows you to remember important information that could help to protect you at some point in the future. However, encoding of emotionally significant memories can become maladaptive where stress becomes chronic or is traumatic. Stress can also bring about impairment in memory retrieval and in working memory.

The seahorse, the chief executive, and the emotional almond

The prefrontal cortex (chief executive), the hippocampus (seahorse), and the amygdala (emotional almond) are the key players involved in both the stress response and in memory function. Chronic stress impacts on plasticity in all three structures, enhancing it in the amygdala but impairing it in the prefrontal cortex and the hippocampus, leading to an interesting pattern of behavior that could impact on making brain-healthy life choices.

The first studies on the impact of stress on cognitive function came about after it was noticed that pilots during the Second World War who were highly skilled during peacetime often crashed their planes during the stress of battle due to mental errors. Early research that tried to understand this phenomenon showed that stress impaired performance on tasks that required complex, flexible thinking but improved performance on easier, habitual, or well-rehearsed tasks. The types of tasks impaired by stress are those that rely on the prefrontal cortex.

Under non-stressful conditions your prefrontal cortex intelligently regulates your behavior through a series of extensive connections with other brain regions, including the amygdala and the hippocampus. Your prefrontal cortex allows you to make decisions, judge situations, and determine appropriate behavior in social situations. It also allows you to outthink faster and stronger opponents or competitors. Through neural networks it supports working memory, allowing you, for example, to maintain information about an event that has just occurred while you access information from your past experience and use the combined information to inform your decisions, regulate your behavior and thinking, monitor your emotions, and modify your emotional behavioral responses.

Reflective versus reflexive

I love speaking in public. The pleasure that I get from imparting information to an audience hungry for knowledge is immense. But for many people even thinking about speaking in public can cause them to break out in a sweat. Public speaking when perceived as a stressor impairs working memory and cognitive flexibility, but it actually improves classical conditioning[21] of negative stimuli as well as hippocampal memory.

When the amygdala activates stress pathways under conditions of psychological stress it leads to the release of high levels of noradrenaline[22] and dopamine,[23] which impair prefrontal cortex regulation but enhance amygdala function.

Your behavior patterns switch from slow, thoughtful prefrontal responses to rapid, reflexive, emotional responses.

While switching the brain from thoughtful, reflective regulation by the prefrontal cortex to more rapid, reflexive regulation by the amygdala and other subcortical structures might save your life if you are in acute danger and need to act fast, it can have negative effects when you need to make choices that require thoughtful analysis and the ability to control or inhibit your more impulsive behaviors or reflexive responses.

Loss of control during stress can lead to relapse of a number of behaviors that impact negatively on brain health, such as smoking, drinking alcohol to excess, overeating, and drug addiction. Prolonged stress can also leave us vulnerable to depression. The molecular events that rapidly flip the brain from reflective to reflexive responding may also contribute to the degenerative changes associated with Alzheimer's disease.

Stressful events can have a profound effect on learning and memory. Stress hinders the updating of memories with new information so that there is a shift from flexible cognitive learning to more rigid, habit-like behavior.

A delicate balance

In addition, chronic stress disrupts the relationship between the prefrontal cortex and the hippocampus that we need for flexible thinking and memory consolidation. It also enhances fear and anxiety and impairs working memory. The activity of neural networks and growth of neural connections increases in the amygdala but in the hippocampus activity reduces and there is a loss of neural networks in both the hippocampus and prefrontal cortex. BDNF (Miracle-Gro) is increased in the amygdala but decreased in the hippocampus.

Chronic stress strengthens structures in your brain that promote the stress response and weakens the structures that provide negative feedback on the stress response, impairing your ability to control or switch it off.

Stress-induced structural changes to the hippocampus require several weeks of stress exposure, but changes in the prefrontal cortex can begin after just one week of stress. Thankfully, animal research suggests that the changes that occur in the prefrontal cortex and in the hippocampus are reversible, which is a good incentive to start managing stress.

Altering the architecture

Recovery from stress-induced changes in neural architecture after the stressful event can be viewed as a form of neuroplastic adaptation.

Resilience in the face of stress is a key aspect of a healthy brain. However, persistence of these changes when stress ends indicates failed resilience.

Stress and the aging brain

Stress in early life and chronic stress during adulthood can reduce the brain's resilience and increase its vulnerability to subsequent exposure to stress, which can impact negatively on the brain as it ages. However, scientific research suggests that physical exercise and engaging in cognitively demanding tasks can help to protect the brain against the damage caused by stress and help to maintain neuronal plasticity during aging.

Chronic or repeated exposure to stress has its highest impact on the brain structures that are undergoing age-related changes in later life and on those that are developing at the time of the stress exposure in young individuals. In later life, neurogenesis and neuronal survival rate in the hippocampus are negatively affected by stress.

Stress plays a key role in brain aging, so managing stress is critical to maintain a youthful brain. Changes brought about by physiological aging can interact with chronic stressors, leading to greater vulnerability of the brain when faced with elevated levels of stress hormones and metabolic challenges, as well as reduced resilience to subsequent exposures to stress. The prefrontal cortex and the hippocampus are most affected by age-related brain-volume loss and by Alzheimer's disease and other dementias.

Assessment: Stress Frequency

Indicate the frequency at which you experience the signs/symptoms of stress in the table overleaf to get a sense of the impact of stress on your life and behavior.

	Never	Once a month	Once a week	2–3 times a week	Every day	1–2 times a day	All the time
Forgetfulness/ absentmindedness							
No sense of humor							
All work and no play							
Unhealthy eating habits							
Feelings of loneliness or isolation							
Not sleeping or sleeping fitfully							
Headaches							
Feeling irritable							
Tense muscles							
Feel tired or fatigued							
Feeling bored							
Feeling depressed							
Short-tempered, angry or hostile							
Worried							
Anxiety							
Feelings of panic							
Upset stomach							
Feeling restless, itchy, uncomfortable in your own skin							

Your responses will help you to to answer Question 1b in Part Two of this chapter (Brain Health Goals: Stress).

COMMON SIGNS OF STRESS

Learning how to recognize the signs and symptoms of stress will help you to take action to reduce harmful effects and minimize the likelihood that stress will become chronic.

Feeling forgetful?

Absentmindedness is a common sign of stress. Stress interferes with the ability to learn and remember and can affect the ability to remember to do things in the future, like taking regular medication or meeting a friend for lunch. Concentration and sleep can also be impacted by stress. Sleep disturbance and impaired concentration can then, in turn, impact negatively on memory function.

All work and no play?

If stress is prolonged or chronic it can trick us into narrowing focus to the extent that we fail to set aside time for physical exercise or other leisure activities such as hobbies, music, art, or reading, or even just socializing with family and friends. It's not difficult to see how it can impact negatively on brain health.

Lost your sense of humor?

Stress can steal our sense of humor, robbing us of our ability to see the funny side of life. Laughter is the ultimate stress buster and humor helps us to cope with the unthinkable. Laughter actually reduces levels of the stress hormone cortisol. Stressed individuals with a strong sense of humor become less depressed and anxious than stressed individuals with a less well-developed sense of humor.

Unhealthy eating habits?

Stress can lead to overeating and unhealthy food choices. In the short-term stress can suppress appetite, but in the longer term if stress becomes chronic and is left unmanaged cortisol can increase your appetite and increase your motivation to eat. Caffeinated drinks and foods high in sugar can contribute to stress by ramping up your amygdala.

Not sleeping or sleeping fitfully?

Stress can make it difficult to fall asleep and stay asleep. When your body is in balance cortisol is secreted into your blood in a predictable twenty-four-hour rhythm. Chronic stress can interfere with this.

Anyone who has experienced disturbed sleep due to stress knows what it's like to be woken in the middle of the night with too much cortisol sloshing around, only to fall asleep in the early morning unable to rouse yourself when your alarm goes off because your cortisol levels are depleted.

Feeling lonely?

When stress is overwhelming it is very tempting to shut others out of our lives because we need time alone to think. We might also avoid others in order not to inflict our stress-induced crankiness or irritability on them. The effort required to be with friends and family can feel like an added stressor, so we end up isolating ourselves at the very time that we should be seeking social support. Isolating ourselves in this way can actually make things worse and have profound effects on our physical, mental, and brain health.

Persistent stress can have adverse and enduring effects on brain function and behavior. Staying socially engaged is critical for brain health and persistent or severe stress can impact on our social behavior. When we are going through a stressful time we can withdraw from social interactions, which, as you will learn in the next chapter, are vital for brain health. Stress can make us irritable and even hostile to others.

> **No-Brainer**: Manage stress to protect your hippocampus and prefrontal cortex from shrinking.

Summary

- Optimal amounts of stress keep you motivated, allowing you to adapt to change to become more resilient.
- Psychological stress refers to the extent to which a person perceives that their demands exceed their ability to cope.
- Stressors can be real or imagined—even a tenuous thought or a faint emotion can trigger the stress response and lead to changes in your cognition, your mood, your behavior, and your health.
- Severe or prolonged stress can negatively impact your behavior and your brain function, including your ability to learn and remember.

- Chronic stress can disrupt your sleep, which is vital for brain health.
- Stress steals resources that would be better used for attention, learning, and memory.
- With chronic stress your behavior patterns switch from a slow reflective response pattern to rapid reflexive emotional responses. This might save your life in circumstances of acute danger but can have negative effects when you need to make choices that require thoughtful analysis and the ability to control or inhibit your more impulsive or reflexive behaviors.
- Stress quite literally changes the structure of your brain and how it functions.
- Chronic or repeated exposure to stress has its highest impact on the brain structures that are developing and on those that are undergoing age-related changes in later life.

Brain Changers: What You Can Do

The goal is to find your personal stress sweet spot. You don't want too much or too little stress but just the right amount for you—a bit like Goldilocks. You can test out your stress boundaries in a variety of ways. You could just do whatever it is that is causing you stress: ask that special person in your office out on a date, go for a job interview, or go to the theater on your own. Or you can go for incremental and gradual exposure to your stressor, such as overcoming your fear of drowning by learning to swim, but do so slowly, starting with dipping a toe in the water rather than jumping in at the deep end.

TEN PRACTICAL TIPS TO MANAGE STRESS

1. Be excited.
2. Be active.
3. Be present.
4. Be positive.
5. Be balanced.
6. Be realistic.

7. Be practical.
8. Be interested.
9. Be happy.
10. Be connected.

1. Be excited

Stress is a natural part of living. It keeps us motivated and allows us to adapt to change and to become more resilient. Life would be boring and static without challenge, uncertainty, and novelty. What would life be like if we never went on that first date, attended that job interview, or made that speech? If we manage our stress and stressors well by preparing properly and seeking support when needed, stressful events can be an opportunity for personal growth and achievement.

We still feel the fear and often want to flee, but when we come out the other side we reap the rewards, we feel invigorated, alive, proud— we can also look back on and learn from the experience. A small shift in perspective from fear to excitement can make a huge difference. Next time you get that wobbly feeling in your gut, try naming it as excitement rather than stress—the feelings are almost identical. It's your choice. Remember, courage grows out of fear.

2. Be active

Exercise and physical activity reduce stress and release endorphins that make us feel good. Physical activity has direct benefits on brain structure and function (Chapter 7). Exercise also improves heart and mental health, reducing levels of depression and anxiety. Making time for daily exercise is a great way to manage stress and is an effective way to improve mental alertness, concentration, and overall cognitive function.

Physical activity can also improve sleep, which can suffer during times of stress. Spending most of the day sitting without moving can increase anxiety levels, so make time to move around during the day. Even five minutes of aerobic exercise can stimulate anti-anxiety effects.

3. Be present

When we are stressed it can be difficult to keep focused on the task at hand. Being present and focused on doing what we are doing while we are doing it is a natural antidote to stress-induced absent-mindedness.

Being "in the moment" also helps us to stay away from negative thoughts or memories that can cause anxiety, stress, and depression. Rooting awareness in the body—such as feeling the soles of your feet connect with the ground while walking, or focusing on breathing in and out—can tie you closer to the present moment.

4. Be positive

Negative thinking can be both a source and a consequence of stress and is a common symptom of anxiety. Practicing positive thinking not only helps reduce stress but also has very real brain-health benefits (Chapter 8). Try writing out your negative thoughts. The simple act of putting them on paper may release your brain from having to remember them.

5. Be balanced

Your body likes regularity and needs internal balance to maintain health. Stress can disrupt this balance in a way that can have serious consequences for health. Eat and exercise regularly. Go to bed at a regular hour each day and allow your body time to rest and recuperate after stressful events.

Set boundaries to ensure you have a good balance between work and the rest of your life. Switch off email notifications and only check your messages at predetermined times. If you can, treat work as a place, not a thing. Make time for hobbies, socializing, and relaxing.

6. Be realistic

Be realistic about what you can achieve. Recognize when good enough is better than perfect. Also, be realistic about what those around you, such as work colleagues, employees, friends, and family, can achieve.

7. Be practical

We all know what it's like to run around the house first thing in the morning frantically searching for keys—it's just another stressor on top of a long list of stressors that you can do without when you are already running late.

Simple things like making a single place for all of the important things in your life—such as keys, wallets, and glasses—can help reduce stress. No more mad panics in the morning.

Keep a stress journal to identify your own personal triggers, and also identify and avoid situations that feed your stress.

8. Be interested

Sometimes stress fools us into narrowing focus to the things that stress us. We put the blinkers on and forget to do things that interest us. Hobbies seem unimportant and even a frivolous waste of time, especially when we have so little of it and so much to do. But engaging with hobbies that interest us is a wonderful stress-buster that can give a real sense of achievement when feeling understimulated and indeed when you're feeling overwhelmed by other aspects of life. Hobbies can challenge your brain and provide opportunities for learning and fun, by allowing you to make use of some of your best skills. They have the capacity to totally engage you to the point where you lose track of time and find distance from the stressors in your life.

9. Be happy

My favorite stress-busters are smiling and laughter. Laughing with other people is rewarding, it boosts bonding and reduces stress and anxiety. Although the neural basis of laughter is not well understood, laughter is thought to act a bit like an anti-depressant, raising serotonin levels in the brain and elevating your mood. When your brain is overloaded with information it looks for biofeedback from your body. By smiling you can send signals to your brain to trigger the release of brain chemicals that can help to dissipate stress and anxiety. You can read more about how smiling benefits brain health in Chapter 8.

10. Be connected

Resist the temptation to withdraw when stressed. Seek support from friends, family and, if necessary, health professionals. Choose wisely who you will spend time with—you need support, not someone who will add to your stress. You can read more about the benefits of social connection in the next chapter.

STRESS—PART TWO

Goals—Action Plan—Personal Profile

Set your goals, devise your action plan, and create your personal profile for Stress.

Brain Health Goals: Stress

Answering the following questions using the information from your Life Balance Log, your Stress Log and your assessment scores will help you to set stress-management goals to boost your brain health.

Q1. Average stress level

a) Base your answer on your response to the *Quick Question: Average Stress*

My average stress level is: Low ☐   Moderate ☐   High ☐

b) Based on the information in *Assessment: Stress Frequency*
The stress frequency table should give you a snapshot of the impact that stress is having on your life and your behavior. If you experience signs/symptoms every day or all of the time or are experiencing a high number of symptoms you may be chronically stressed and need to manage your stress better.

Stress Goal No. 1

I would like to manage my stress better ☐

No action required: I am happy with how I manage stress ☐

Q2. Perception of stress

a) Based on how you usually feel, answer the following:

I see life's challenges as opportunities:
    Rarely ☐   Sometimes ☐   Usually ☐

I focus on things that I can control:
    Rarely ☐   Sometimes ☐   Usually ☐

I focus on things that I cannot control:
    Rarely ☐   Sometimes ☐   Usually ☐

b) Based on your total score on the *Assessment: Perceived Stress*

My perception of stress is: Low ☐   Moderate ☐   High ☐

Stress Goal No. 2

I want to change how I perceive stress: Yes ☐ No ☐

No action required: I am happy with how I perceive stress ☐

Q3. Daily stress

**Based on the information from your *Assessment: Stress Log*
complete the table below.**

Indicate whether you would like to focus your energy on changing the
stressor or changing your response to the stressor.

Stressor	Can control	Cannot control	Change stressor	Change response

Stress Goal No. 3

I want to change my response to stressors I cannot control:
Yes ☐   No ☐

No action required: I'm happy with how I respond to stressors beyond my control ☐

I want to remove or change stressors that I can control:
Yes ☐   No ☐

No action required: I'm happy with how I manage stressors ☐

Q4. Life balance

I'm not a fan of the term "work/life" balance as it somehow implies that work is negative and a source of stress. It is very individual. For many, work is rewarding and a source of great joy. The aim is not to spend more or less time in work, it is to ensure that you have balance across activities that you enjoy, that give you just the right amount of stress, sleep, and exercise, while leaving room for laughter and time outdoors.

Based on your *Assessment: Life Balance Log*, complete the table below.

	Rarely	Sometimes	Usually
I am happy with the number of hours I work			
My work gives me a sense of fulfillment			
I am happy with the number of hours I spend with family and friends			
I am physically active at least five days per week			
I am happy with the number of hours I spend on hobbies and interests			
I am happy with the amount of time I spend outdoors			
Smiling and laughter are a part of my personal life			
Smiling and laughter are a part of my work life			
I am happy with the number of hours I spend sleeping			

Stress Goal No. 4

I want to change how I invest my time to achieve better life balance: Yes ☐   No ☐

No action required: I am happy with how I invest my time ☐

Completing the table below using the information from your Stress Goals will help you to characterize your current healthy habits and prioritize any stress habits that need fixing. Tick the box that applies then enter any items that need fixing into the Brain Health Action Plan on the next page.

	Healthy	Needs fixing	Priority*
How I perceive stress (PSS score)			
How I respond to stressors			
Daily physical exercise			
Time spent connecting with others			
Time spent working			
Time spent on hobbies/interests			
Time spent smiling and laughing			
Number of hours sleep per night **			
Time spent in nature			
Time spent on technology			
Organization and preparedness			
Caffeine consumption**			
Sugar consumption			
Other			

* High, medium, or low

** Base your response on the Sleep Log that you completed in Chapter 3.

Brain Health Action Plan: Stress

Enter your stress habits that need fixing into the Brain Health Action column in the table below. Indicate whether the action is attainable with relative ease in the short term (quick fix) or will require more time and effort to achieve (long term). The ten tips that you have just read should help you to break each action into practical steps. Prioritize the actions in the order you would like to work on them (1 = tackle first). *You will find a completed sample in the back of the book.*

Brain Health Action	Order	Steps	Quick fix	Long term

Personal Profile: Stress

Using your scores in the **Brain Health Goals: Stress** section as a guide, complete this table. Indicate whether your scores are healthy, borderline, or unhealthy. From that you can determine whether your current pattern of behavior is a brain-healthy asset or a risk that could compromise your brain health and make you vulnerable to dementia in later life. Finally, indicate the aspects that you would like to fix, improve, or maintain and prioritize them for inclusion in your bespoke Brain Health Plan in Chapter 9.

Aspect	Healthy	Borderline	Unhealthy	Asset	Risk	Maintain	Improve	Fix	Priority
Stress level									
Perception of stress									
Daily stress									
Life balance									
Total									

100 Days to a Younger Brain

PROGRAM DAYS 8–14: MANAGING STRESS

You should now have a clear understanding of your current stress patterns, your personal goals, and the actions that you need to take in order to manage stress to benefit your brain health. You will combine your stress profile with the other profiles that you will create as you complete this program to build your overall Brain Health Profile in Chapter 9. You will also select at least one of your stress actions to add to your overall Brain Health Plan.

100-DAY DIARY

You can record the steps that you are taking toward your program goals in the 100-Day Diary at the back of the book. For example:

- I was much more realistic about how much work I could get through today.
- I only checked my emails once in the morning and once in the afternoon.
- I ate my lunch outside today instead of at my desk.
- I switched off my computer and phone notifications at 6 p.m. today.

You can also celebrate your healthy habits by recording them in your 100-Day Diary.

5

Stay Social, Go Mental

"It is good to rub and polish our brain against that of others."
Michel de Montaigne

SOCIAL AND MENTAL—PART ONE

Humans are funny creatures really, when you think about it. Our logic can be quite flawed. We blame cognitive decline on aging rather than on the fact that we tend to frontload activities that are beneficial to brain health, such as learning and social engagement, into childhood, youth, and early adulthood. We are social beings and being social stimulates the brain to the benefit of brain health and mental health. When we live a life that is socially integrated and engaged we experience slower cognitive decline and are less likely to get Alzheimer's disease. The evidence is mounting that social engagement helps to maintain cognitive functioning.

Social interactions are often intertwined with other activities that also influence brain health, including learning and cognitively stimulating leisure activities that occur in the company of others. Education can build reserves at any point during life, yet as a society, generally speaking, we focus our education efforts mainly on children, teens, and young adults. Some people are fortunate to have occupations that continue to stimulate the brain and provide opportunity for challenge, but sadly by middle age many of us are coasting along on autopilot, happy to take the easy road.

You'll find plenty of practical ideas for engaging your brain and your buddies to benefit your brain health in this chapter. Completing the assessments will give you a better understanding of your social needs and mental activity levels to help you to make changes to boost your brain health. You will use this information to create your personal social and mental profile, set goals, and devise a social and mental action plan in Part Two of this chapter. First, let's explore the neuroscience behind why we need to welcome people, challenge, novelty, and learning into our daily lives.

Quick Question: Social

How often do you feel isolated from others? ___

Where 1 = hardly ever; 2 = some of the time; 3 = often

Brain Gains: Why Do You Need to Keep Your Brain Active?

Our survival depends on us being social. We are instinctively predisposed to maintain proximity to other humans and to avoid isolation. Our survival depends on reciprocal relationships. We form bonds that provide mutual aid. Social bonds keep us safe and allow us to reproduce. Humans tend to perish in isolation. People with more social ties are less likely to develop dementia or cognitive impairment in later life than people with fewer social ties. People with more social ties have better health, are less depressed, and live longer.

BEING SOCIAL AND SOCIAL BEINGS

The brains of humans, and indeed primates in general, appear to be particularly sensitive to social influences. In primate species there is a relationship between the size of their social group and the relative volume of their neocortex. As a species humans are highly skilled socially. The human brain evolved alongside these skills. The complexities required for social living, including the ability to predict behavior and outsmart others, may have led to the expansion of the human brain and to the elaboration of neural systems within the brain. Social cognition is fundamental to functioning within the social world that we inhabit, allowing us to get along with other people and see other points of view. Disturbances in social cognition, such as reduced empathy, abnormal social behavior, and difficulty taking the perspective of others, can be an early feature of neurodegenerative disorders.

Social engagement refers to our interaction with others in our environment. It includes all of our social interactions, our social activities, our social networks, and our functional and emotional social supports. Your social environments help to shape your brain. Your social interactions with friends, family, colleagues, neighbors, and strangers bring about plastic changes in your brain, affecting both its structure and how it functions. Answer the following questions to assess your social connectedness.

Assessment: Social Connectedness

1. Are you currently?

    Married ☐   Living with a partner as married ☐
    Single (never married) ☐

    Separated ☐   Divorced ☐   Widowed ☐

2. Do you participate in any groups, such as senior center, social or work group, religious-connected group, self-help group, or charity, public service, or community group? Yes ☐   No ☐

3. How often do you go to religious meetings or services?

    Never or almost never ☐   Once or twice a year ☐
    Every few months ☐

    Once or twice a month ☐   Once a week ☐
    More than once a week ☐

4. How many close friends do you have, people with whom you feel at ease or can talk to about private matters?

    None ☐   1 or 2 ☐   3–5 ☐   6–9 ☐   10 or more ☐

5. How many close relatives do you have, people with whom you feel at ease or can talk to about private matters?

    None ☐   1 or 2 ☐   3–5 ☐   6–9 ☐   10 or more ☐

Ques.	Social connectedness	Score
1	Relationship status Married or living with a partner as married (1) All others (0)	
2	Participation in any groups Yes (1) No (0)	
3	Participation in religious meetings or services Once or twice a month or more frequently (1) Every few months or less frequently (0)	
4 & 5	Close friends and relatives 2 friends or fewer and 2 relatives or fewer (0) All other scores (1)	
	Total social connectedness score (max score = 4)	

*Answers to Questions 2 and 3 should be mutually exclusive.

What your score means

A score of 0 or 1 being the most isolated category, scores of 2, 3, or 4 represent increasing levels of social connectedness.

Transfer your score to Question 3, Part Two of this chapter (Brain Health Goals: Social and Mental).

As a species our interactions with others shape the neural circuits that underlie our social behavior. Socially engaged lifestyles and stimulating environments are associated with the growth of new neurons and with an increase in the density of synapses. Social activity increases brain volume and leads to more efficient use of brain networks. *Just ten minutes of social interaction can boost your brain performance.*

The social brain

You employ complex brain activity and demonstrate incredible cognitive dexterity whenever you engage in social interactions, enabling you to understand other people's words and actions, read their emotions, filter your own thoughts, and formulate appropriate responses. Often you will do this while also carrying out another activity, such as walking or balancing a drink in one hand while reaching for a canapé with the other.

The complex network of regions in your brain involved in social interaction and social cognition are collectively known as the social brain. This network is involved in numerous social processes that allow you to recognize other humans—their faces, their gestures, and their emotions—communicate with others, explain your own behavior, understand and predict the behavior of others, and evaluate the beliefs, intentions, desires, dispositions, and actions of others.

Some social processes are automatic and unconscious and therefore beyond your conscious control. However, thanks to your prefrontal cortex, you do have conscious control over many of your social behaviors. For example, you can stop yourself from blurting out an honest but hurtful comment about your best friend's new haircut.

Being able to regulate yourself in this way allows you to preserve important relationships and keep your emotions and actions within the realms of socially acceptable behavior. Lack of sleep, stress, aging, injury, brain disease, and some disorders can compromise your brain's ability to self-regulate in this way, as many of us have learned the hard way when we say the wrong thing or fail to filter when we are over-stressed or over-tired.

While specific areas of your brain become active when you engage socially or even when you think about people or try to make sense of social relationships, your social brain doesn't operate in isolation. Areas of your brain involved in processing non-social information also play a part. Social and emotional behavior are closely linked and structures in your brain that process emotions are also involved in your social behavior. Social engagement requires the coordinated action of brain areas distributed across your brain. These areas are specialized in processing social information, non-social information, and emotional information.

Content and context

Which areas are activated at any one time is very much dependent on content and context. For example, faces activate your fusiform face area (FFA), which is a part of the brain located at the back of your temporal lobe. However, in order to recognize the emotions represented through facial expression, other areas of your brain that decode emotional signals need to be activated. If the expression on the face that you are looking at is one of fear, your amygdala will be activated. If the expression is one of disgust or pain, an area of your brain called the anterior insula will be activated. Emotions are very powerful social signals that allow you to respond to others and shape how others respond to you.

The most recently evolved part of your brain, the neocortex, can be referred to as your "thinking brain." The oldest part of your brain that sits atop your spinal cord is known as the brain stem or the reptilian brain. Your limbic brain, also known as your midbrain or emotional brain, is sandwiched between the two. You need your reptilian brain to control the functions most basic to your survival, such as your heartbeat, breathing, and digestion. Your midbrain handles love, anger, guilt, and other emotions, while your neocortex, which contains your frontal lobes, is capable of interpreting and formulating extremely complex and sometimes conflicting information.

As you interact socially these reptilian, emotional, and thinking brains work together via multiple operating systems, sometimes in coordination and sometimes in conflict, depending on the context. Resisting a decadent chocolate dessert is an example of the systems in conflict — you want to eat the cake (basic function), it will make you feel good (emotion), but you want to fit into that new outfit so that you look good at your friend's wedding (thinking). So you don't eat the cake!

Mirror neurons

Your brain also contains cells called mirror neurons, which are not only activated when you complete an action yourself but also when you view the action being completed by someone else. These brain cells mirror the action that you see and are crucial to how you perform your own actions and how you monitor and interpret those of other people.

Essentially, these mirror neurons allow you to put yourself in someone else's shoes. These simulations can occur so fast that you are unaware of them.

Areas in your brain such as your premotor cortex simulate the actions that you observe and this simulation also triggers activity in areas of your brain involved in emotion, such as your amygdala. This tightens the link between imitation of the action and identification with the person that you observe carrying out the action. That's why you experience similar emotional and physiological reactions when you witness someone else experiencing pleasure or pain, as if you were the person involved. It also might explain why you find yourself wincing when you witness someone sustain an injury or crying when your favorite contestant on *The Voice*, *American Idol*, or *Dancing with the Stars* wins or is eliminated.

While you watch your favorite sport, the motor system in your brain is activated just as if it was you kicking that ball, returning that serve, or swinging that golf club. Then when your emotion centers are triggered you also feel the ecstasy and the agony of victory and defeat. This allows you to understand the mental states of others, interpret and predict their actions and intentions, and empathize with them.

Social engagement

We are not entirely sure why a socially engaged lifestyle positively impacts on cognitive function. It is of course possible that changes in levels of social engagement may occur as a consequence of decline in cognitive function rather than the other way around. Poorer cognitive function might result in reduced ability to function socially, or the stigma of cognitive decline or feelings of embarrassment about memory loss might lead people to withdraw socially. Reduced mobility or even fear of falling while out and about can also limit opportunities for social stimulation in older people.

What we do know for sure is that human connection is inextricably linked with our cognitive function, our brain health, our physical health, our mental health, and our emotional well-being. It is possible that cognitive function might benefit because social support buffers the negative effect that chronic stress can have on the brain.

Social factors might also influence cognitive outcomes because social engagement may make positive health behaviors more likely. The idea here being that in the absence of friends and family we are likely to either neglect or indulge ourselves to the point that it damages our health, increasing our risk of cognitive decline. However, there is mounting evidence that social engagement is a form of cognitive stimulation that contributes to cognitive outcomes via the building of cognitive reserve.

MENTAL STIMULATION

In addition to social engagement, cognitive reserve is linked to carrying out mentally stimulating or cognitively demanding tasks, occupation, and the level of education an individual has attained. Education is the most broadly and consistently successful cognitive enhancer, better even than drugs or sophisticated technology. I mentioned in Chapter 1 that as the world's population of older people grows the number of older adults with dementia is predicted to increase to 132 million by 2050. While there are some early onset forms, dementia is mainly a disease of later life so it follows logically that if you have more older people in a population you will also have more people in that population living with dementia.

However, in the United States and in some countries in Europe an optimistic trend of declining age-specific dementia risk has emerged in recent years, which may moderate the increase in dementia that is predicted to accompany the growing number of older adults. The growth in levels of educational attainment in successive generations together with more widespread and successful treatment of cardiovascular risk factors are considered key in this welcome decline in dementia risk.

Investing in education is like investing in cognitive reserve. A direct consequence of this investment is the development of compensatory neural circuits within the brain that build capacity to withstand damage, thereby delaying the onset of dementia and compressing cognitive impairment closer to end of life, just like Peter in the introduction. Answer the following questions to assess your education/occupation profile.

Assessment: Education and Occupation

A. Formal education

How many years in total have you spent in formal education?___

Include primary school, secondary school, university—they don't have to be continuous years. So if like me you went to university as a mature student, add those years to the time you spent in school when you were younger.

Less than eight years score = 0

More than eight years score = 1

Formal Education Score ___

Transfer your score to Question 2a, Part Two of this chapter (Brain Health Goals: Social and Mental).

B. Formal academic

What is your highest academic qualification?_____

For example, PhD, Master's, Bachelor's degree, Diploma.

Circle the score in the table below that corresponds to your highest academic qualification.

Level / Qualification	Score
Advanced doctoral degree/fourth-level degree (e.g., PhD)	20
Completed Master's degree	18
University/college graduate with Bachelor's degree	16
Diploma involving two or more years at university/college	14
Completed final second-level exams/graduated high school	11
If you left education without any formal qualifications your score is the actual number of years you spent in formal education	

Formal Academic Score ___

Transfer your score to Question 2b, Part Two of this chapter (Brain Health Goals: Social and Mental).

C. Lifespan occupation

Present

Indicate your current employment situation?

☐ Retired

☐ Employed

☐ Self-employed

☐ Unemployed

☐ Long-term sick or disabled

☐ Looking after the home or family or both

☐ In education or training

Lifespan

Thinking back over your adult working life, indicate in the table below how many years you have spent in each of the occupation categories listed. Record the number of complete years you were engaged in each professional category. Leave blank if you never worked in a particular category.

Indicate whether your job mainly involved you working alone (solo) or working with and/or interacting with people (social).

The categories are somewhat artificial but they give a rough indication of occupational levels of mental and social activity involved. If you are unsure, choose the category that most closely matches the level of mental activity/intellectual challenge of the job that you had.

When you add together the years under each category they should add up to the total number of years you have spent in employment.

If you have never been employed your answer will be zero.

Occupation category	Years	Social	Solo
Low-skilled or manual work			
Skilled manual work			
Skilled non-manual work			
Professional occupation			
Highly intellectual or responsible occupation			
Total years in employment			

Multiply the number of years spent in the occupational category by the number indicated in the column below. Then add the scores for each category together to get your total Lifespan Occupation Score.

Profession	Years	Multiply by	Score
Low-skilled manual—mainly solitary		1	
Low-skilled manual—mainly social		1.25	
Skilled manual—mainly solitary		2	
Skilled manual—mainly social		2.25	
Skilled non-manual—mainly solitary		3	
Skilled non-manual—mainly social		3.25	
Professional		4	
Highly responsible/intellectually demanding		5	
Total Lifespan Occupation Score			

Lifespan Occupation Score ___

Transfer your score to Question 2c, Part Two of this chapter (Brain Health Goals: Social and Mental).

Lifelong learning

Fringe benefits of educational investment may include more cognitively stimulating occupations, higher economic status, and better health behaviors. Given its relevance to brain health, education can't just be for school, it's got to be for life. Lifelong learning is vital for brain health. The protective effect of cognitive reserve inferred by education, occupation, and mental stimulation cuts the risk of developing dementia almost in half. Longer years in education are associated not only with decreased risk of dementia but also with greater brain weight and so potentially greater brain reserve.

There is no relationship between years in education and neurodegenerative or vascular pathologies in the brain. Education doesn't offer protection against developing neurodegenerative and vascular pathology in your brain but it does seem to mitigate the impact that that pathology has on the clinical expression of dementia. *Education doesn't prevent your brain from becoming diseased but it does seem to lessen the impact the brain disease has on cognitive functioning, most probably through brain and cognitive reserve.*

Invest in leisure

Reading, hobbies, and artistic or creative pastimes can also help to protect against cognitive decline. One study that well illustrates this examined whether engaging in cognitively stimulating leisure activities (reading, writing, crosswords, board/card games, discussions, and playing music) in later life could affect the trajectory of memory decline.

Over the course of the study 101 of the 488 participants developed dementia. In the people who had developed dementia, each additional day that they engaged in the leisure activities delayed the onset of accelerated memory decline for two months. Engaging in stimulating leisure activities seems to boost resilience and allow people to cope with or compensate for Alzheimer's brain changes for longer before manifesting severe memory loss.

Furthermore, this positive effect was independent of education level. Essentially, participants reaped the reward irrespective of whether they had left school early or had high levels of educational attainment. That is particularly meaningful when you realize that after age, low educational attainment is the single biggest risk factor for dementia. Complete the table on the next page to assess your leisure activities.

Assessment: Leisure

Frequency: Indicate the frequency at which you engage with any of the activities listed: daily = 5, once or twice a week = 3, once a month or less = 1, rarely or never = 0.

Form social: If you engaged in the activity with others, enter the frequency score under the social column as well. If you engaged in the activity alone, enter the frequency under the solo column.

Form mental: If the activity challenges you, enter the frequency score for the activity in the challenge column as well. If the activity involves learning, enter the frequency score for the activity in the learning column as well. If the activity involves doing something new, enter the frequency score for the activity in the novelty column as well. If the activity involves none or only some of the above, leave the columns blank accordingly.

Leisure activity	Frequency	Social	Solo	Challenge	Novelty	Learning
Example: Reading	5		5			5
Example: Cinema	2	2				
Go out to the cinema, plays, and concerts						
Attend classes, lectures, or further education						
Travel for pleasure						
Work in the garden, in your home, or on a car						
Read books/magazines for pleasure, including on devices						
Listen to music or radio						
Play games, e.g., cards, chess, crosswords, puzzles, and games (computer/video) involving strategy or problem solving						
Go to the pub						
Eat out of the house						
Participate in sport, activities, or exercise						
Visits to or from family or friends, either in person or talking on the phone						
Volunteering						
Creative activities						
Other hobbies and interests						
Visit museums, galleries, exhibitions						
Total Leisure Score:						

What your score means

Frequency: If you scored 0 for nine or more activities, you may be at greater risk of developing dementia and need to increase the number of leisure activities that you participate in. If you engage in six or more leisure activities at least once a month, you are at less risk of developing dementia.

Transfer your total scores for Challenge, Learning and Novelty to Question 1, Part Two of this chapter (Brain Health Goals: Social and Mental).

Transfer your total scores for Social and Solo to Question 5, Part Two of this chapter (Brain Health Goals: Social and Mental).

Challenge, novelty, and learning

While everyday leisure activities are clearly beneficial, you can really ramp up the brain-health benefits by challenging yourself and by learning and experiencing new things. Challenging your brain stimulates the connections between neurons, essentially promoting neuroplasticity. It may help to fight off decline in mental functions such as memory and it may offer some protection—not only against diseases like dementia that occur in later life but also against diseases like multiple sclerosis that affect people in their twenties.

Your plastic brain can be bent and reshaped as you learn and make new memories but that mesh of neurons needs to be challenged if it is to reorganize itself effectively. Stretching yourself a little, doing things beyond your comfort zone, or pushing yourself into situations that require you to cope with challenges will change your brain chemistry, impacting positively on your mood and your brain function.

Reward

In your frontal lobes the neurotransmitter dopamine facilitates the flow of information from other areas in your brain. Dopamine neurons in your brain become activated when something good happens unexpectedly. The satisfaction that you experience from mastering a challenge will lead to the release of dopamine, making you feel good, more positive and less depressed. Dopamine is released when we expect or receive a reward such as food or music, or when we surmount a challenge. Dopamine also tells your brain that whatever you experienced is worth getting more of and so can help you to change your behaviors in ways that will allow you to attain more rewarding experiences and achieve your brain-health goals.

Novelty

Your dopamine system is most responsive to novel and unpredictable rewards. Your brain thrives on regularity and predictability, but paradoxically the need for predictability drives your brain to seek novelty. The more information your brain has about your environment the better it will be able to compare experiences and predict the probability of certain outcomes. Being rewarded by novel events better positions you to gain insight from your environment. Novelty also causes your brain to release noradrenaline, which helps to form new brain connections. Novelty—experiencing new things, new people and new situations—is a critical element of neuroplasticity.

When you engage your brain in mentally stimulating activities you strengthen your synapses. For your brain to benefit you need to constantly challenge yourself. Routine activities don't challenge your brain, you need to push yourself to the next level, try something different, or learn something new.

Learning, the brain changer

Learning is like a powerful brain-changing drug generating new brain cells, enriching brain networks, and opening new routes that your brain can use to bypass damage. Lifelong learning results in a range of positive outcomes, including reduced risk of social isolation, increased mental and social activity, and improved quality of life and well-being.

Lifelong learning also benefits your brain health, reduces your risk of developing dementia, and increases your chances of continuing to live independently in later life. The human brain was built for learning and change so that we can adapt to an ever-changing world. **Your brain confers on you the ability to do tomorrow what you couldn't do today.** Learning is not just for the young. Learning is for everyone.

Learning is for living and learning is for life.

> **No-Brainer**: Novelty is a critical element of neuroplasticity. Make room in your life for new people and new experiences.

Brain Drains: What Happens When Your Brain Is Deprived of Social and Mental Stimulation?

As you age the rule is "use it or lose it." Neglecting social and mental activities leads to disuse of the brain, which in turn is linked to atrophy of cognitive function. Unused branches in your brain are pruned, while regularly used connections are strengthened. This is a natural process, but as you age neurons that are left out of action through lack of use become damaged and die.

If you've ever tried to learn a famous speech, a presentation, or a long poem, you will know that it is quite a testing task. In a way it's like beating a path through an overgrown hedge. It's tough at first but through repeated use or repetition you lay down a proper track through the hedge. Eventually you form an indelible memory like a path through the brambles.

If you become an expert in one skill, be it rapping or rhyming, music, dance, or design, entire regions of your brain may be reshaped. Some changes can take years but change can be swift, too. If you are blind-folded, within just two hours extra touch signals are rerouted via the area of your brain that normally deals with vision. Eventually, much of the area could switch function. The brain does not allow parts to lie fallow—blind people use the vision department of their brain for hearing.

Reroute, reuse, rewire

Rerouting is a key strategy of damaged brains. Rather than try to repair a broken network, neurons will sometimes go around a blockage and make do with what is available to get a circuit back up and running. If you discovered a large boulder in the middle of your well-trodden path through the brambles, would you try to move the boulder or would you start working on a new path to go around it to take you to your ultimate destination?

In animal studies we see that brain cells beside a damaged area adopt new functions and shapes that allow them to take on roles from their damaged neighbors. This has important implications for rehabilitating people who sustain brain injury from stroke, or who lose function through diseases such as multiple sclerosis. If, for example, a person does not practice a movement lost to brain injury or stroke, the damaged brain cells and surrounding tissue are starved of stimulation and may die off. We now know there is great scope for brain compensation and recovery with the right practice and training, at the right time. Therein lies the hope and the hard work.

The cost of social stress

Your brain and your body are fully integrated with each other via mutually interactive biochemical and neural regulatory circuits, which include immune, hormonal, and neural components. The physiological operations that occur while you go about your daily business of behaving and being you come about as your brain and body work together. These operations can only be understood in the context of your environment, including the physical and social environment in which you are interacting. The social and the physiological are inextricably linked.

Regardless of what is going on in the outside world, whether your external environment is hot or cold, in crisis or calm, you need to maintain a stable internal environment throughout your body and brain and within each of your cells. The hypothalamus in your brain is responsible for this system-wide maintenance of optimal conditions (homeostasis) that is critical for your health and your survival. But every time your body responds to a stressor (such as extreme cold, illness, or a fright), to restore homeostasis there is a physiological cost to making that adjustment. Unlike the physical stress of lifting weights in the gym, which ultimately builds muscle and strengthens bones, persistent social stress, such as prolonged social isolation and chronic loneliness, increases wear and tear throughout your body and your brain.

Isolation and loneliness

Our tendency to engage in social activities primarily with people the same age as us is preventing us from fully benefiting from the positive outcomes associated with social engagement. In part this is because, and there is no nice way to say this, when we socialize only with people our own age our social circle will diminish in later life with each passing year as old friends die off.

Of course, there is value in socializing with our age peers as we share life references and life stages, but we also need to consciously seek opportunities to enrich our social circles with people younger and indeed older than us, so that as a society and as individuals we continue to reap the benefits of being socially integrated at all stages of life.

People with less social participation, less frequent social contact, and more feelings of loneliness have an increased risk of developing dementia. To put this in perspective, the risk associated with loneliness and social isolation is comparable in size with well-known risk factors for Alzheimer's disease, including physical inactivity, low educational attainment, mid-life high blood pressure, type 2 diabetes, smoking, and depression.

The health behaviors of lonely young people, including their exercise and eating habits, are no worse than those of their socially embedded age peers. However, over time this changes, so that by middle age the health habits of lonely people become worse. Lonely older people are less likely to engage in physical exercise than socially contented older people. In addition, lonely older adults exercise less each day than their socially contented counterparts. Lonely older people are also more likely to take a higher percentage of their daily calories from fat than socially contented older people.

Being alone and feeling lonely are not the same thing

American philosopher Paul Tillich says that we created the word loneliness to express the pain of being alone and the word solitude to express the glory of being alone. Feeling lonely and being alone are not the same thing. We can be alone but not feel lonely. When it comes to social contentedness we all have different needs.

Feelings of loneliness and social isolation are very individual and not always directly related to the size of our social networks. Some people need constant contact, frequent social interaction, and large social circles, while others feel socially contented with one or two deep and meaningful social interactions a couple of times a month.

Feelings of loneliness emerge when there is a mismatch between what we need and what we have in terms of the quality and quantity of our social relationships. We can feel lonely, alienated, and isolated even when we are with others. Being among family and friends does not automatically satisfy our need for social intimacy.

If you have felt lonely it just means that you are human. While some of us are more predisposed to feelings of loneliness, most of us will experience loneliness at some point or indeed at several points in our lives. Some common times when people experience loneliness are:

attending college for the first time; becoming a new mum; when newly divorced or recently retired; when bereaved or caring for a spouse with dementia; when living alone; when unemployed; and even when working from home.

Feeling lonely makes us less likely to employ our social skills, and over time our social skills diminish through lack of use, so we may come across as socially awkward. But we do not become lonely because we are socially awkward, rather, we can become socially awkward through social isolation and loneliness, which is assessed in the questionnaire below.

Assessment: Loneliness

When answering the questions, remember there are no right or wrong answers, so be completely honest. When answering it is best to think of your life as it generally is now (we all have some good or bad days).

	Hardly ever	Some of the time	Often
How often do you feel that you lack companionship?			
How often do you feel left out?			
How often do you feel isolated from others?			

Score your answers as follows for all questions:

Hardly ever	Some of the time	Often
1	2	3

What your score means
Adding together your scores from all the questions will give you a possible range of scores from 3–9.
Scores from 3–5 are generally taken to mean not lonely.
Scores from 6–9 are generally taken to mean lonely.
Transfer your score to Question 4, Part Two of this chapter (Brain Health Goals: Social and Mental).

Why do we feel lonely?

The sensations associated with loneliness evolved because they contribute to our survival as a species. Loneliness is a painful experience.

We use the word pain to describe a variety of unpleasant sensory and emotional experiences. Pain information is transmitted to the central nervous system. Pain is a signal that we cannot ignore. Pain tells us to get out of this situation now. People born with insensitivity to pain are easily injured and tend to die at an early age. Just as physical pain evolved to protect us from physical dangers, the unpleasant social pain of loneliness evolved to protect us from the dangers of being isolated. Loneliness is an unpleasant feeling that we try to avoid.

A variety of biological mechanisms have evolved that capitalize on what psychologists refer to as "aversive signals" to motivate us to engage in behavior that is essential to our survival. For example, the sensation of hunger, triggered by low blood-sugar levels, motivates us to eat, and the sensation of thirst motivates us to drink. Loneliness in small doses is adaptive because it spurs us on to seek social contact, but when we ignore the signal, loneliness can become chronic and this represents a serious threat to our general health and to our brain health.

Loneliness is a killer

Social isolation—and especially perceived isolation—negatively impacts on health through effects on the brain, on the physiological stress response, on sleep, on blood pressure, on inflammatory processes, and on the immune system. People who are lonely, who live alone, or who are socially isolated have an increased risk of early death. This is most likely a consequence of the impact that social deficits have on diseases that ultimately lead to death.

Being a member of a social species comes with benefits (protection and assistance) and costs (risk of infection and competition for food and for mates). From an evolutionary perspective, being isolated from our social group can be perilous, making us vulnerable to predators. Feelings of loneliness act as a biological warning, an alarm bell, motivating us to take action to avoid isolation.

However, the brain also switches into self-preservation mode when we feel socially isolated. Changes occur in the brain, which make us more alert to danger, more distrustful and less empathetic toward others. Ironically, this can make us more likely to isolate ourselves socially. If we remain lonely, over time our social skills become eroded through disuse.

Loneliness experienced over long periods may act as a chronic stressor, increasing the activity and number of neural connections in our brain's fear center (the amygdala), putting us on high alert and keeping us in high self-preservation mode. Loneliness doesn't just make you feel unhappy, it can make you feel unsafe and interfere with sleep, which can have a knock-on effect on health and well-being.

The release of cortisol and "fight or flight" activity in the sympathetic nervous system[24] can also overstimulate the inflammatory response and suppress our immune response. The effect of stress on the immune system can also be indirect—if we try to cope with loneliness, for example, by drinking or smoking. Chronic stress can also lead to shrinking of the prefrontal cortex, which plays a key role in regulating our social behavior, allowing us to empathize with and make sense of the world. Loneliness is also associated with poor sleep quality and high blood pressure, both of which impact on cognitive function and our risk of developing dementia.

Loneliness is a serious problem that has deep roots in our biology as well as our social environment. We need to be aware that some of our brain's automatic and unconscious responses may color our perception of the world, disabling our ability to empathize and tricking us into seeing threat where there is none.

Choose to connect

But it is equally important to remember that while some of these responses are automatic and unconscious we do have some cognitive control. We can make choices. We can consciously take action to routinely engage more socially, and if we see others who have become isolated we need to help to reintegrate them in a way that takes account of the fact that their brain has undergone changes that makes them fearful, less empathetic, and possibly socially inept.

> **No-Brainer**: Use it or lose it. Seek out social interaction and mental stimulation.

Summary

- Living a life that is socially integrated and engaged is associated with slower cognitive decline. People with more social ties are less likely to develop dementia or cognitive impairment.
- Social interactions bring about structural and functional plastic changes in the brain.
- Interactions with others shape the neural circuits that underlie our social behavior.
- Socially engaged lifestyles and stimulating environments are associated with the growth of new neurons and with an increase in the density of synapses.
- Social activity increases brain volume and leads to more efficient use of brain networks.
- Social engagement may be a type of cognitive stimulation that contributes to positive cognitive outcomes via the building of cognitive reserve.
- Education is the most broadly and consistently successful cognitive enhancer, better even than drugs or sophisticated technology.
- Education doesn't prevent your brain becoming diseased but it does seem to lessen the impact that the disease has on cognitive functioning.
- Engaging your brain in stimulating leisure activities may allow you to cope with Alzheimer's brain changes for longer before they manifest as memory loss.
- Challenging your brain promotes neuroplasticity.
- Novelty—experiencing new things, new people, and new situations—is a critical element of neuroplasticity.
- Lifelong learning results in reduced risk of social isolation.
- Learning is like a powerful brain-changing drug that generates new brain cells, enriches brain networks, and opens new routes that the brain can use to bypass damage.
- Use it or lose it. As you age, neurons that are left out of action through lack of use become damaged and die.

- Persistent social stress, such as prolonged social isolation and chronic loneliness, increases wear and tear throughout your body.
- The dementia risk associated with loneliness and social isolation is comparable in size with well-known risk factors for Alzheimer's disease, including physical inactivity, low educational attainment, mid-life high blood pressure, type 2 diabetes, smoking, and depression.
- Loneliness makes you feel unsafe.
- Loneliness is a killer.
- If you have felt lonely it just means that you are human.
- While some responses associated with loneliness and social isolation are automatic and unconscious, we do have some cognitive control. We can engage our cortex to make choices to support social integration.

Brain Changers: What You Can Do

The goal is to find the right level of social engagement to meet your personal needs and keep your brain stimulated but not overloaded. What constitutes beneficial mental stimulation is also very individual. The key is to introduce challenge, novelty, and learning based on where you are at now. Focus on incremental progress toward a longer-term goal; attaining small achievable targets gives you a sense of achievement and the motivation to keep learning and challenging yourself. Make sure you socialize with people who make you feel good about yourself and select activities that you enjoy doing and set goals for yourself that mean something to you.

TEN PRACTICAL TIPS TO STAY
SOCIALLY AND MENTALLY ACTIVE

1. Volunteer.
2. Be selective.
3. Cultivate a vibrant and varied social circle.
4. Reach out online.
5. Start small.

6. Welcome novelty.
7. Love learning.
8. Embrace education.
9. Create challenge.
10. Combine benefits.

1. Volunteer

Volunteering is a great way to increase social engagement, increase social interactions, and support a stimulating lifestyle. Volunteering may actually help you to live longer and improve your brain health. People who volunteer are happier, less depressed, and report better health than those who don't.

Volunteering at a homeless or animal shelter, with a charity organization, a local community group, or sports club can be a good place to start. If it's been a while since you were socially connected, engaging in small talk about the weather, the game, the animals, or the soup can be calming and can help to bring about the positive changes in your brain chemistry to move you away from fear and give you safe opportunities to practice rusty social skills.

2. Be selective

When seeking opportunities to increase social interaction, focus on the things that you like and enjoy doing. This will increase the likelihood of connecting with others with similar interests. Quality matters—be selective about who you socialize with. It is important that the relationships are pleasant and meaningful for you.

Not all social relationships are positive, and the last thing you want is a social relationship that undermines your brain health through stress. Unsupportive social ties might also present barriers to your efforts to improve your own health behaviors and outcomes. Be aware of the "social contagion" of negative health behaviors whereby your personal risk of obesity is increased by having an obese spouse or friend, and having risk-taking friends can, for example, increase your alcohol consumption.

It is important to have at least one trustworthy and reliable confidant in your life with whom you feel you can communicate regularly. For many that confidant is someone that they have known since childhood, or it might be a spouse or life partner. It might be worth considering fostering additional relationships of this kind as unfortunately in later life we can lose that person to ill-health or death, and while it will never be possible to replace that special someone it is important to have a trustworthy, supportive listening ear.

3. Cultivate a vibrant and varied social circle

With each successive generation we are becoming increasingly time poor and the demands of modern life can fool us into seeing socializing as a luxury pushed to the bottom of our to-do list. After reading this chapter I hope that you will see that social interaction is fundamental to brain health and must be factored into your life.

Try to cultivate a group of family, friends, neighbors, or work colleagues that you can regularly engage with to exchange thoughts, ideas, worries, plans, hopes, and dreams. Make mealtimes a shared occasion and an opportunity for social engagement in your own home with your family, at a local community center that offers a lunch service, or combine catching up with friends over lunch or dinner.

Interest groups, clubs, community groups, classes, and courses are great ways to meet people of all ages. Try to seek opportunities to engage with and nurture friendships with people of different ages. Check yourself for prejudices as you chat, and dismiss these thoughts in favor of openness and a willingness to discover more about the person than their age.

4. Reach out online

Internet use is associated with decreased feelings of loneliness, higher levels of both social connectivity, and perceptions of social support. If friends and family are flung far and wide the Internet can help you to stay connected through email, messaging, online social networking, and Skype. You can also use digital technology to expand your social networks or reignite relationships with old friends.

In terms of addressing social isolation and loneliness, social networking works best as a springboard to offline interaction rather than a replacement for face-to-face connection. However, research shows that older adults engaged in online communities benefit from intellectual stimulation and emotional support. Online social engagement may help to compensate for lost relationships and provide a personal space free from stress.

5. Start small

If you or a loved one currently feel socially isolated or have persistent feelings of loneliness it's probably wise to take it slowly. Stick a tentative toe in the social water—do it safely, don't dive right in. Because of heightened perception of threat you need to experiment in a safe environment. It may also help to acknowledge the hypervigilant processes in your brain that may make you see threat where there is none. The same process may also mean that you will initially encounter difficulty seeing other people's point of view.

Work on switching your perspective so that you expect the best rather than the worst in others. This will take time but if your first response is to see the negative in a social interaction, take a moment to question your response and see whether you can reframe it in a positive light. Be patient with yourself and with your brain. Be realistic, you will need to allow time to retrain your brain, especially if you have been chronically lonely.

Start small—hold a door open for someone or share a smile with someone. Venture a nod, a wave, or a hello with a neighbor or someone in your local shop or supermarket.

If you or a loved one have mobility, transport, safety, or other issues that prevent or make it difficult for you to get socially connected, consider connecting with online communities or reaching out to local community groups or befriending organizations. Your local social services or primary health care center may be able to help you to connect with these organizations or community groups.

6. Welcome novelty

Accepting change into your life can be a challenge in itself, but your brain will benefit if you can find ways to do this. If you always take the easy road you can become stuck in a rut and your brain won't be prepared for challenges that may lie ahead. You also risk becoming bored, apathetic, and depressed. Be innovative, experiment, there are lots of simple ways to introduce new things into your life. The following list is really just to get you thinking.

- Listen to a genre of music that you have never listened to before.
- Read a section of the newspaper that you don't usually read, or start a book from an unfamiliar genre.
- Tune in to a different radio station.
- Take time to read about cultures or viewpoints that are novel to you.
- Take your hobby to the next level: move from quick crosswords to cryptic, cook or bake more complicated recipes, learn a new carpentry skill, add new songs to your repertoire...
- Try a new restaurant or order something different from the menu in your favorite restaurant—preferably something you've never tasted before.
- Try walking a new route to work. Change your jogging route. Take up a new sport or try a new technique.
- Visit new places, find opportunities to meet new people, become a tourist in your own city.

7. Love learning

As children we are driven by curiosity. We ask questions and if that doesn't satisfy our curiosity we ask some more. We interact with the world using all of our senses. We try to figure things out ourselves. When we see something new we want to try it out. Unfortunately, for many of us the joy of discovery gets lost to learning by rote and studying for tests and exams. As a consequence we often associate learning with negative emotions, such as unpleasant stress, failure, or even boredom. If we do succeed academically our satisfaction comes from the reward of exam grades, qualifications, awards, or promotions rather than the joy of learning.

If you have forgotten the true joy of learning it may be time to reignite your curiosity. Make a list of things that have always fascinated you and promise to learn more about them. Be curious about the world around you. Try looking at things through the eyes of a toddler or a visitor from outer space. Allow yourself the time to wonder how things work or question why we do things the way we do. Ask questions of yourself, of others, and of the *grandmaster*, Google. Let yourself be amazed at everyday things. Avoid the cynical shrug, the "whatever," or the "who cares." Test assumptions.

Don't limit your world to the familiar. Afford yourself the opportunity to encounter the unfamiliar. Diversify your interests. Don't assume that your viewpoint or worldview is correct, question it and inform it. Become curious about other viewpoints, worldviews, cultures, etc. Allow yourself to be curious about and amazed by the world and the people around you.

8. Embrace education

Make a personal commitment to lifelong learning. It can be formal or informal, online or in person, for personal fulfillment or professional advancement. Your chances of success are greater if it is something that interests you, something that you enjoy and derive pleasure from. From a personal perspective I can recommend returning to formal education. I understand that returning to full-time education is unlikely to be an option for most people, due to financial or time constraints, but there are so many options to explore and many that are entirely free.

There are hundreds of free Massive Online Open Courses (MOOCs) available from a variety of sources. The courses appeal to multiple tastes and interests; you can study languages, literature, politics, business, culture, science, psychology, nature, history, creative arts, tech, coding, and much, much more. Many MOOCs are social learning platforms, which means that the courses enable learning through conversation, so people taking the course engage with each other and with the educators through online forums. The online lessons, which usually require a modest time investment (two to three hours per week) take a variety of forms (videos, text, quizzes etc.).

Whether you read up on a topic that interests you, take a night class, join a book club or a historical society, or study for a degree, just make a commitment to lifelong learning.

9. Create challenge

The key is to set yourself challenges that stretch you but don't push you too far. You want to step just outside your comfort zone. This is something that will be very individual. You are more likely to succeed if you choose something that you enjoy doing or that involves a goal you are motivated to achieve. You can simply choose a new activity that challenges the way you think.

Alternatively, if you already engage in a cognitively stimulating activity, why not try to push yourself to the next level? If you play a musical instrument, challenge yourself with a new complex piece that pushes you to the boundaries of your musical ability, commit yourself to a performance or consider learning another instrument. You can apply similar principles to any skills, arts, creative pursuits, sport, hobbies, leisure, or intellectual activities.

There is a lot of hype around brain training games. So it is important to mention that a recent consensus statement on the brain training industry from the scientific community states that, while some training produces statistically significant improvement in the practiced skill, claims made promoting brain games are frequently exaggerated and at times misleading. That's not to say that they won't be shown to work at some point in the future but at this point in time it is important to acknowledge that more research is needed and findings need to be replicated by independent researchers with no financial interest in the product.

Any new experience that involves mental effort is likely to bring about changes in the neural systems that support the acquisition of that new skill. So changes will occur with computer games but they will also occur with any novel mentally stimulating activity such as learning a new language, learning how to juggle, learning to play a new musical instrument, or finding your way around a new town on holiday. The consensus report also echoes my own feelings that time spent playing games is time not spent engaging in other activities such as socializing, exercising, and reading, that benefit physical, mental, and brain health.

10. Combine benefits

Why not pick a hobby or skill that you can learn with someone else or one that involves social interaction? Joining a choir or a book club will not only stimulate your brain but will also bring extra benefits for your mental health. Being part of a group or having an activity partner might add to the fun and also help to keep you motivated. Consider challenging yourself by taking up a new sport; the learning involved will stimulate your brain. If you take up a team sport you will experience the added social benefit. On top of that the physical exercise will benefit both your brain health and your heart health.

In the next chapter you can read more about why looking after your heart health is vital for brain health.

SOCIAL AND MENTAL—PART TWO

Goals—Action Plan—Personal Profile

Set your goals, devise your action plan, and create your personal profile for Social and Mental.

Brain Health Goals: Social and Mental

Answering the following questions will help you to set social and mental activity goals to boost your brain health.

Q1. Leisure

Based on your total score on *Assessment: Leisure*

Challenge Score ___ Learning Score ___ Novelty Score ___

There are no cut-off scores or recommended daily doses for mental stimulation. However, we do know that your brain will benefit if your leisure activities challenge you and involve learning and opportunities for new experiences.

Take another look at your **Assessment: Leisure** table on page 120 to see whether you could use your leisure time to better benefit your brain. Consider engaging in activities more regularly or taking on new activities from the list that you engage in less often or not at all.

Mental Goal No. 1

I want to engage in more leisure activities: Yes ☐ No ☐

I want to incorporate
more challenge: Yes ☐ No ☐
more novelty: Yes ☐ No ☐
more learning: Yes ☐ No ☐
into my leisure activities

No action required: I am happy with the number
of leisure activities I take part in ☐

I feel challenged by my leisure activities ☐

I regularly have new experiences in my leisure time ☐

I am constantly learning throughout my leisure time ☐

Q2. Education and occupation

Base your answers on your *Assessment: Education and Occupation* sections A (Formal Education), B (Formal Academic), and C (Lifespan Occupation).

a) Formal Education Score _____
b) Formal Academic Score _____
c) Lifespan Occupation Score _____

Mental Goal No. 2

I want to engage with formal education: Yes ☐ No ☐

I want to engage with informal education: Yes ☐ No ☐

I want to take a class or training course in my leisure time:
Yes ☐ No ☐

I want to take a class or training course at work:
Yes ☐ No ☐

I want to spend more time educating myself:
Yes ☐ No ☐

No action required. I am as educated as I want to be:
Yes ☐ No ☐

Q3. Social connectedness

Base your answer on your score from the *Assessment: Social Connectedness*

My social connectedness score is: Low ☐ Moderate ☐ High ☐

Social Goal No. 3

I would like to increase my level of social connectedness:
Yes ☐   No ☐

No action required: I am happy with my level of social connectedness ☐

Q4. Loneliness

Base your answer on your score on *Assessment: Loneliness*

I am: Lonely ☐   Not lonely ☐

I feel this score is an accurate reflection of how I feel: Yes ☐   No ☐

Social Goal No 4.

I want to do something about my feelings of loneliness:
Yes ☐   No ☐

No action required: I don't feel lonely ☐

Q5. Balance social and solo

Base your answers on the *Assessment: Leisure*

a) My leisure activity social score _____

b) My leisure activity solo score _____

The aim here is to have a good balance between social and solo activities.

Social Goal No. 5.

I want my leisure activities to involve more:

Social engagement: Yes ☐   No ☐

Solitary leisure activities: Yes ☐   No ☐

No action required, I am satisfied with:

The social levels of my leisure activities ☐

The level of my solitary leisure activities ☐

Completing the table below using the information from your Social and Mental Goals will help you to characterize your current healthy habits and prioritize any social and mental habits that need fixing. Tick the box that applies then enter any items that need fixing into the Brain Health Action Plan on the next page.

	Healthy	Needs fixing	Priority*
Activities that challenge me mentally			
Activities that involve new experiences			
Activities that involve learning			
Social activities			
Solo activities			
Social connectedness			
Loneliness			
Other			
Other			

* High, medium, or low

Brain Health Action Plan: Social and Mental

Enter your social and mental habits that need fixing into the Brain Health Action column in the table below. Indicate whether the action is attainable with relative ease in the short term (quick fix) or will require more time and effort to achieve (long term). The ten tips that you have just read should help you to break each action into practical steps. Prioritize the actions in the order you would like to work on them (1 = tackle first). *You will find a completed sample in the back of the book.*

Brain Health Action	Order	Steps	Quick fix	Long term

Personal Profile: Social and Mental

Using your scores in the **Brain Health Goals: Social and Mental** section as a guide, complete this table. Indicate whether your scores are healthy, borderline, or unhealthy. From that you can determine whether your current pattern of behavior is a brain-healthy asset or a risk that could compromise your brain health and make you vulnerable to dementia in later life. Finally, indicate the aspects that you would like to fix, improve, or maintain and prioritize them for inclusion in your Brain Health Plan in Chapter 9.

Aspect	Healthy	Borderline	Unhealthy	Asset	Risk	Maintain	Improve	Fix	Priority
Leisure									
Education									
Occupation									
Connectedness									
Loneliness									
Balance social/ solo									
Total									

100 Days to a Younger Brain

PROGRAM DAYS 15 AND 16: GETTING SOCIALLY AND MENTALLY ACTIVE

There is no log to complete this week so just use the two days to complete the questionnaires in this chapter and check out local and online activities or courses that interest you. When you are putting together your plan, keep in mind that it's good to push yourself beyond your comfort zone.

You should now have a clear understanding of your current social and mental activity patterns, your personal goals, and the actions that you need to take to benefit your brain health. You will combine your social/mental profile with your other profiles that you will create while you complete the program to build your overall Brain Health Profile in Chapter 9. You will also select at least one of your social/mental actions to add to your overall Brain Health Plan.

100-DAY DIARY

You can record the steps that you are taking toward your program goals in your 100-Day Diary at the back of the book. For example:

- I had dinner with my family this evening.
- I chatted with another shopper in line at the supermarket.
- I researched local volunteering opportunities.
- I read a section of the newspaper I wouldn't normally read today.
- I started reading a classic novel that I bought in a charity shop today.
- I listened to a science podcast today.
- I read online about Aztec culture/learned why stars twinkle today.

You can also celebrate your healthy habits by recording them in your 100-Day Diary.

6

Love Your Heart

*"Our bodies are our gardens to which
our wills are gardeners."*
William Shakespeare

HEART—PART ONE

When it comes to life, do you follow your head or your heart? Your heart health and brain health are closely connected—if you look after your heart your head will follow. Over the last twenty-five years there has been a huge increase in cardiovascular risk factors, including diabetes, high blood pressure, and obesity. These risk factors usually emerge in mid-life due to unhealthy life choices such as smoking, physical inactivity, and diets high in sugar and salt—mainly due to processed or fast foods. These factors are also linked to increased dementia risk.

On a positive note, in recent years we have seen considerable improvements in treatment for and control of cardiovascular risk factors, including high blood pressure, high cholesterol, and high blood sugar. These have improved population heart health and this has had a knock-on effect that makes our brains healthier, too. Such improvements have reduced the incidence of heart disease and together with increased levels of education they are also considered responsible for the trend of declining age-specific dementia risk that has emerged in recent years.

This chapter is packed with practical tips and tests to help you gain a clearer understanding of your current heart health and risk factors. The Food Log will help you make adjustments to transform your heart health to benefit your brain health.

You will create a personal heart profile, set goals, and devise a heart action plan in Part Two of this chapter, but first let's go to the neuroscience to find out how your heart health and brain health are closely connected and what can happen if this relationship breaks down. If you look after your heart your brain will benefit. Read on, it's time to show your heart some love.

Quick Question: Heart

Have you ever been told that you have high blood pressure?
Yes ☐   No ☐   Don't know ☐

Brain Gains: What Has the Heart Got to Do with Brain Health?

Your brain uses more energy than any other organ in your body. That energy is delivered to your brain by your blood. Every time your heart beats, blood carrying oxygen and nutrients essential for brain health and survival is pumped to your brain through a rich network of blood vessels. Damage to this vascular system can have catastrophic consequences for you and your brain. Heart disease is responsible for one in four deaths in the United States and UK every year—that's pretty shocking when you consider that 90 percent of cardiovascular disease is preventable. In the context of brain health, cardiovascular risks aren't just associated with heart disease and death, they are closely linked to cognitive impairment and dementia. In fact, about a third of all cases of dementia can be attributed to vascular issues.

Your brain relies very heavily on your heart and vascular system to do its job efficiently and effectively. Brain atrophy (wasting) is closely related to cardiovascular disease, obesity, and diabetes. Making unhealthy choices can lead to narrowing of your blood vessels and, over time, hardening of the arteries in your body and in your brain. A build-up of fatty plaques in the arteries or stiffening of the arteries not only leads to heart disease but can also disrupt the supply of oxygen-rich blood to your brain cells. Without an adequate supply of oxygen and nutrients, your brain will begin to malfunction and your cognitive function will deteriorate. If your brain is suddenly deprived of oxygen you will have a stroke. In addition to the immediate impairment to brain function caused by stroke, one in three people who survive a stroke will go on to develop dementia, so it is really important to know your numbers. Completing the assessment below will help you to do this.

Assessment: Heart Health

Blood pressure

Record your blood pressure ___ / ___
Don't know ☐

If you don't know your blood pressure, aim to get it checked this week by your doctor or local pharmacist. Many pharmacies now offer a free service.

If you have been told by a medical professional that you have high blood pressure or hypertension, how are you managing your blood pressure? _____

Transfer the results of your medical test into Question 1, Part Two of this chapter (Brain Health Goals: Heart).

Cholesterol

Has a doctor ever told you that you have abnormal or unhealthy cholesterol levels?
Yes ☐　No ☐

If yes, how are you managing your cholesterol?_____

Record your cholesterol/HDL ratio_____
Don't know ☐

Transfer the results of your medical test into Question 2, Part Two of this chapter (Brain Health Goals: Heart)

Diabetes and blood sugar

Tick the box if a doctor has ever told you that you have any of the following:

Type 2 diabetes ☐   Type 1 diabetes ☐   Any other type of diabetes ☐
Pre-diabetes (metabolic syndrome) ☐

Have you ever been told by a doctor that you have abnormal or
unhealthy blood sugar levels? Yes ☐   No ☐

If yes, how are you managing your blood sugar levels? _____

_____

Transfer the results of your medical test into Question 3, Part Two of this chapter (Brain Health Goals: Heart).

Since the 1990s we have learned a huge amount about brain function from functional magnetic resonance imaging (fMRI). This non-invasive brain-imaging method has afforded us unprecedented access to the detailed inner workings of the human brain. Every one of your thoughts, feelings, and actions has been made possible through the electrical and chemical signaling of the billions of brain cells inside your skull. When you wiggle your big toe there is an increase in the electrical activity in the areas of the brain that generate that movement. To feed this increased demand, more oxygen is delivered to that area by your blood.

Information gleaned from fMRI scanning is pretty cool but it can't tell us everything. Sometimes findings can be difficult to interpret because certain areas that "light up" on fMRI have more than one function. But for the purpose of the topic at hand we can say that when you engage in a cognitive activity like reading or playing the piano, the areas of the brain involved in that activity will need to receive more oxygen to support the increased electrical activity.

Blood pressure

Blood pressure is particularly important for brain health. Your heart works like a pump; when it clenches it is using pressure, like water in a garden hose, to push blood through your arteries around your body and to your brain. Your heart uses this pressure and enough hose to go around the world twice to make sure that every single part of your body and your brain are serviced.

You don't want your blood pressure to be too high or too low. You want it to be just right. If it's too low you might feel light-headed and might faint or fall. But if it's too high you probably won't have any symptoms at all. And, to be honest, you may look well on the outside but, on the inside, high pressure is causing damage to your arteries and your heart is placed under huge strain. If left unchecked, over time, this kind of damage can disrupt the delivery of vital supplies to your brain. A healthy diet can help to reduce your risk of high blood pressure. It can also promote brain health and reduce your risk for heart disease, high cholesterol, and diabetes. In addition it can prevent unhealthy weight gain.

Brain fuel

Your brain requires a constant supply of fuel. That fuel comes from the food that you eat and what you eat directly affects your brain function and its structure. Foods that will save your heart also pay dividends upstairs, so you can eat your way to a better brain. The phrase "you are what you eat" counts for your brain, too! More accurately, you are what you eat, drink, and inhale.

Your brain is made up of 73 percent water. It is a thirsty organ because your brain needs to be kept hydrated to function properly. If you were to dehydrate a brain (don't try this at home!) you would find that the constituent ingredients of your dried brain soup are fats, proteins, amino acids, minerals, vitamins,[25] and glucose. Each of these macronutrients (fat, protein, and carbohydrates) and micronutrients (vitamins and minerals) impact on brain development, brain functioning, energy, and mood.

Assessment: Weight

Has a doctor told you that you are:

Obese ☐   Overweight ☐   Underweight ☐

Body Mass Index (BMI): *Weight _____kg Height _____cm*

BMI = _____(weight ÷ (height x height))

Waist measurement: _____

Transfer your measurements into Question 4a, Part Two of this chapter (Brain Health Goals: Heart).

Assessment: Food Log

On Days 17 to 23, keep a **Food Log**. Write down everything you eat no matter how big or small. If you can, note the salt, sugar, and fat content, too. Try to complete the log as you go. Use an app if you prefer—there are also some great alcohol trackers online. Be as specific as you can in terms of portions and try comparing your daily intake with the food pyramid guidelines (see government health information websites). Day 17 of your 100-Day Program will be Day 1—the first morning you begin the Food Log. *You will find a completed sample in the back of the book.*

	Day 1	**Day 2**	**Day 3**
Day (e.g., Mon)			
Breakfast			
Lunch			
Dinner			
Snacks			
Water			
Fluids			
Alcohol			
Comments			
Fat			
Salt			
Sugar			
Cigarettes			

Use the information in this Food Log to answer Question 4b, Part Two of this chapter (Brain Health Goals: Heart).

Day 4	Day 5	Day 6	Day 7

Fats

Omega-3 fatty acids are critical for maintaining the health of your brain cells. Your body can't make omega-3 fatty acids so you must get them from foods (fatty fish, nut oils, and some plants). You probably already know that these so-called good fats can help to lower your risk for heart disease, but omega-3 fatty acids are also found in high concentrations in the brain and so are thought to be important for brain performance, memory, and behavioral function, too. They may even be protective against Alzheimer's disease and dementia.

Steroids

Cholesterol is found in your blood. You will probably already be aware that high levels of cholesterol are not good for your heart, but did you know that cholesterol is vitally important for brain function? It is actually a steroid that is essential for human health. It forms the building blocks for hormones, including cortisol, involved in the stress response.

Protein

To function properly your brain and nervous system also need an adequate supply of amino acids, found in protein foods. These amino acids are also like building blocks. In fact, they are the raw materials needed to make neurotransmitters, the chemical messengers that carry signals throughout your brain.

Dopamine, noradrenaline, and serotonin are key neurotransmitters that play a role in cognitive function, including attention, learning, and memory. They also have a role in mood, fear, and pleasure. Amino acids found in the protein that you eat are essentially the precursors of neurotransmitters that play a significant role in your life.

Vitamins and minerals

Your brain benefits from trace minerals, B vitamins, and antioxidants.[26] Minerals such as iron, copper, zinc, and sodium in the right proportions are essential for brain health and cognitive development.

As a child I first learned about iron by watching *Popeye,* whose biceps ballooned each time he downed a can of iron-rich spinach (Google him if you are too young to remember the cartoon). Obviously eating iron doesn't have any such immediate effect on muscles, although it does boost energy levels and increase physical performance. But iron does have many vital functions in your body, including transporting and storing oxygen and energy metabolism. Your brain gets a great boost from iron because your brain needs oxygen to work well. Blood carries vital oxygen supplies to your brain cells, and that process needs iron.

B-group vitamins each have specific effects on brain function. For example, vitamin B12 plays a critical role in making and maintaining the myelin sheaths that protect your axons, ensuring fast and effective transmission of neural signals.

Antioxidants, mainly found in fruit and vegetables, are like damage-limitation specialists; they play an important role in preventing cell damage by neutralizing free radicals that have the capacity to damage and destroy brain cells. The principle antioxidant micronutrients are beta-carotene and vitamins C and E. The body can't manufacture these micronutrients so they must be obtained through diet.

Energy: glucose and oxygen

Your brain is a high-energy consumer and its fuel comes from the food that you eat. Molecules such as sugars, fats, and proteins are high sources of energy because the energy used to form them is stored within the chemical bonds that hold these food molecules together. Your digestive system converts the carbohydrates (sugars and starches) in the food you consume into glucose, which is absorbed by your stomach and small intestines and then released into your bloodstream. Your brain relies almost exclusively on glucose as its energy source.

The billions of neurons in your brain use about one-fifth of the oxygen and glucose circulating in your blood at any one time. While most of this fuel is used for neural communication, about a third is needed for the essential housekeeping that keeps your brain cells healthy and your brain tissue alive.

Neural activity and blood supply

Active regions of your brain consume more energy than inactive regions. Your brain has a very limited capacity to store energy, so the increased energy required by an active brain area is produced locally by glucose and oxygen, supplied by local small blood vessels. Essentially, local vessels expand to allow more blood to reach the specific area to meet the demand for local neural activity.

Your blood needs to deliver just the right amount of oxygen and glucose to the active areas, and the brain has clever built-in systems to regulate this. The cells in your brain and your blood vessels work together to make sure that when you dip your toe in water, write a navel-gazing novel, or go for a swim, the appropriate areas of your brain receive sufficient fuel to support the corresponding brain activity.

Border control

Your brain cells are highly sensitive to chemical changes and function best in a stable environment with efficient waste removal and adequate protection from toxins. The major blood vessels in your brain are lined with a barrier that protects it from substances that might damage it, effectively acting as a border between the blood and your brain. Only those molecules with the right credentials can enter or leave your brain in areas policed by the blood brain barrier. Stroke can disrupt this barrier, leaving the brain vulnerable to invasion by potentially toxic substances. Your cardiovascular system also plays a key role in waste disposal, preventing the build-up of unwanted products of brain activity and metabolism, including beta-amyloid and tau, which are implicated in Alzheimer's disease.

The brain has frequently been described as the most complex structure in the known universe. It is capable of incredible things but it is also very vulnerable and highly dependent on you to provide it with the fuel, water, nutrients, and oxygen that it needs to function. If you mistreat it by ingesting trash or inhaling toxins your brain won't be able to reach its potential and may even struggle to survive. So when you shop for food, shop for your brain.

> **No-Brainer**: Get your blood pressure, cholesterol, and glucose levels checked and follow your doctor's advice to keep them within a healthy range.

Brain Drains: What Happens to Your Brain When You Don't Love Your Heart?

Cumulative exposure to vascular risk factors throughout your life increases your risk for stroke, dementia, and other neurological diseases. Simply put, high blood pressure, high cholesterol, and diabetes are all vascular risk factors that damage cerebral blood vessels, negatively impacting cerebral blood flow, local neural activity, and auto-regulation, leading to neurovascular dysfunction and suboptimal brain health.

Brain attack

A stroke or "brain attack" occurs when the blood flow to an area of the brain is cut off due to blocked, broken, or burst blood vessels. Stroke and the factors that lead to it also play a pivotal role in cognitive impairment and dementia. Stroke is a disease of the blood vessels that service your brain. Despite the fact that 80 percent of strokes can be prevented, stroke remains the leading cause of disability in the United States and UK. *For each minute a stroke is left untreated a patient will lose approximately 1.9 million neurons, 14 billion synapses, and 7.5 miles of neural connections.*

Covert attacks

Many older people sustain vascular brain injuries that are classed as subclinical, silent, or covert. These subtle injuries are caused by tiny blockages to the small blood vessels in the brain, and while these injuries to the brain's vascular system are not severe enough to have the definite or obvious symptoms that you would associate with a stroke that doesn't mean they don't cause damage. They do, and in fact they can be associated with cognitive decline and also increase the individual's risk of having a stroke in the future.

These silent strokes are up to twenty times more common than overt strokes. These kinds of injuries are usually caused by death of brain tissue due to inadequate blood supply to the affected area, damage produced by myelin and axonal loss, and brain micro-bleeds. This type of microscopic damage also raises the likelihood that dementia will emerge at some point in the future.

High pressure

High blood pressure in mid-life is the leading cause of stroke. It is also associated with silent brain injuries in people aged over sixty. If your blood pressure stays high, over time it may increase your risk of developing dementia. Chronic high blood pressure disrupts the delivery service of vital nutrients and oxygen to your brain, which may begin to malfunction. If left untreated, high blood pressure in mid-life can increase your risk of vascular dementia and Alzheimer's disease in later life.

High blood pressure is a warning sign that lifestyle changes are urgently needed.

Depriving your brain of vital nutrients

When it comes to what you eat, drink, and inhale, the choices that you make can have a direct and long-lasting effect on your brain.

Fats

Omega-3 fatty acids are essential for brain function. If you become deficient in omega-3 you will likely experience memory problems, fatigue, mood swings, and depression as well as heart problems and poor circulation. Several studies show that reduced intake of omega-3 fatty acids is associated with increased risk of age-related cognitive decline or dementia, including Alzheimer's disease.

Cholesterol

Your body manufactures its own cholesterol in the liver. In fact, your body can produce all of the cholesterol that it needs to carry out its many essential functions and can generally maintain a healthy level of blood cholesterol so you *don't* need to add foods containing cholesterol to your diet.

Too much cholesterol over time can lead to the narrowing or blocking of the arteries, leading to heart attack or stroke. Consuming trans fats can lead to abnormal cholesterol levels. Eating these fats can impact on your brain health because they can increase your risk of heart disease, stroke, and type 2 diabetes.

Dementia doppelgangers

Some treatable nutrient deficiencies can interfere with cognitive function and mimic dementia.

Vitamin B12

If you become deficient in B12 you may present with symptoms that look a lot like dementia, including a decline in memory, problems making decisions, personality changes, and irritability. Vitamin B12 deficiency also plays a role in stroke risk. Older people are more likely to be affected by B12 deficiency.

As we age changes to our digestive tract may decrease the amount of vitamin B12 that is absorbed. In addition, levels of B12 might also be reduced simply because we tend to eat less in later life. Daily supplementation or vitamin B12 injections are a safe and easy way to address a B12 deficiency and reverse the associated dementia-like symptoms.

Water

Your brain is comprised mainly of water. You need it in your blood to transport oxygen, nutrients, and waste. Generally speaking, we don't drink enough fluids. Age-related changes in thirst sensitivity and kidney function compound the problem of sustained dehydration in older adults. As we get older we feel less thirsty so may drink less. In later life we may experience more frequent urges to go to the bathroom and so we drink less to cut down on bathroom trips. Either way, dehydration can occur and if it is severe it can cause cognitive deficits in short-term memory and can disturb mood. Severe dehydration can look like dementia and sometimes lead to delirium.

Delirium

The symptoms of dementia and delirium can be similar but the latter frequently has a very sudden onset while dementia is characterized by a more gradual and progressive decline. Delirium can usually be traced back to one or more contributing factors, which might include a urinary tract or other infection, a severe illness, or even something like low sodium or a medication. Treating the cause once identified can often reverse the delirium; however, in older adults an episode of delirium may accelerate any underlying decline in cognitive function that pre-exists the delirium. Keeping adequately hydrated and treating infections sooner rather than later is wise.

Glucose

Without enough glucose in the brain, communication between neurons can break down because chemical messengers (neurotransmitters) are not produced. Low glucose levels (hypoglycemia), a complication of diabetes, is associated with poor cognitive function and problems with attention. The frontal lobes are so sensitive to reductions in glucose that altered mental function is a primary signal of glucose deficiency. Diets that are high in sugars promote oxidative stress[27] and have been associated with impaired brain function. Eating a balanced diet rich in vitamins, minerals, and antioxidants can protect the brain from oxidative stress.

Smoking

Oxygen is one nutrient your brain can't live without for more than a few minutes. Smoking raises your heart rate and increases the carbon monoxide levels in your body. Elevated carbon monoxide in your blood causes a build-up of fat on the walls of arteries, narrowing the arteries and decreasing blood flow. While blood is still pumping and delivering blood to brain tissue, the supply of oxygen is hampered by carbon monoxide. Nicotine affects your heart, blood vessels, hormones, and your brain function. Smoking also causes changes in your brain that make you crave more nicotine.

Assessment: Smoking and Alcohol

Smoking

Have you ever smoked cigarettes, cigars, cigarillos, or a pipe daily for a period of at least one year? Yes ☐   No ☐

Smoking status:

Non-smoker ☐   Current smoker ☐

How many cigarettes do you smoke on average each day? _____

Ex-smoker ☐   How old where you when you stopped smoking? _____

For how many years have you been/did you smoke altogether? _____

Smoking harms nearly every organ in the body. It kills people, and it kills brain cells. It has long been associated with poor heart health, cancer, and lung disease. But did you know that smokers have thinner cortices (outer layers of the brain) than non-smokers? The longer you smoke the thinner your cortex gets. You need your cortex to think, to speak, to act, and to process information, so shrinking it through smoking is not smart.

Alcohol

*Base your answers on the information you recorded in your **Sleep Log** in Week 1 and in your **Food Log** this week if these weeks are representative of your normal pattern of alcohol consumption.*

How many units of alcohol do you consume on average each week?_____

How many alcohol-free days do you have on average each week?_____

Do you ever have more than six drinks in one day? Yes ☐   No ☐

Transfer your score to Question 6, Part Two of this chapter (Brain Health Goals: Heart).

No-Brainer: Eat a balanced diet, maintain a healthy weight, keep hydrated, and quit smoking.

Summary

- Your brain is highly dependent on your heart and your blood vessels to deliver the oxygen and nutrients that are essential for the functioning and survival of your brain cells.
- Vascular damage can have catastrophic consequences for you and for your brain. About a third of all cases of dementia can be attributed to vascular issues.
- Blood pressure is particularly important for brain health. High blood pressure can cause damage to your arteries and your heart and over time this can disrupt the delivery of vital supplies to your brain.
- Stroke and the factors that lead to it play a pivotal role in cognitive impairment and dementia.
- What you eat and drink directly affects your brain function and its structure. Your brain is incredibly vulnerable and highly dependent on you to provide it with the fuel, water, nutrients, and oxygen that it needs to function. If you become deficient in omega-3 you will likely experience memory problems. A vitamin B12 deficiency can look a lot like dementia. Chronic dehydration can increase your risk of high blood pressure and stroke.
- Diets that are high in sugars promote oxidative stress, which can lead to heart and blood vessel disorders and neurodegenerative diseases. Eating a balanced diet rich in vitamins, minerals, and antioxidants can protect your brain from oxidative stress.
- Smoking kills brain cells. Smokers have thinner cortices than non-smokers. The longer you smoke the thinner your cortex gets.

Brain Changers: What You Can Do

Lifestyle choices have a hefty say in heart health. There are lots of ways by which you can help to protect your heart to benefit your brain. It's really important to actively monitor and manage your health, so do have your blood pressure, blood sugars, and cholesterol levels screened regularly, especially if you are over fifty.

Whatever your age, you need to be eating a healthy diet, maintaining a healthy weight, and limiting your consumption of alcohol and processed foods to reduce your risk of a cardiovascular event. If you manage your blood pressure, obesity, physical exercise, and diabetes in mid-life you reduce your risk of developing dementia. Managing stress is important, too, and if you are a smoker you need to quit now. You owe it to yourself to take personal responsibility for managing these risks. Loving your heart is one of the greatest gifts you can give to yourself.

TEN PRACTICAL TIPS TO LOVE YOUR HEART

1. Check your blood pressure.
2. Derail diabetes.
3. Shop for your brain.
4. Control your cholesterol.
5. Skip the salt.
6. Hydrate.
7. Watch what you drink.
8. Manage stress and stay connected.
9. Quit smoking.
10. Attain and maintain a healthy weight.

1. Check your blood pressure

One simple thing that you can do is to get your blood pressure tested. High blood pressure (hypertension) has been dubbed the "silent killer" because so many people are unaware that they have it, and because there are no visible symptoms. As a consequence, about half the people with hypertension are undiagnosed. Of those who are aware that they have hypertension, half are untreated and in half of those who are treated their blood pressure remains uncontrolled.

The only way you can find out whether you have hypertension is to get your blood pressure checked. As we get older our blood pressure can sneak up silently so even if it is "just right" now, you need to get it checked regularly to avoid unpleasant surprises in later life.

If you don't currently know your blood pressure, make an appointment to get it tested.

Modifiable risk factors for high blood pressure

Poor diet—consuming a diet high in sodium, calories, sugar, and fats (saturated and trans) increases your risk of high blood pressure. Too much salt leads to fluid retention, which increases pressure. Too little potassium may give rise to too much sodium.

Being overweight or obese—the bigger you are the more blood you need to supply oxygen and nutrients to your tissues, including brain tissue. This increased blood volume increases the pressure on your artery walls and puts extra strain on your heart, increasing your risk of high blood pressure.

Physical inactivity—sedentary people have higher heart rates, and this means your heart has to work harder with each contraction, increasing the force on your arteries.

Smoking—smoking raises your blood pressure temporarily and damages the lining of your artery walls, leading to narrowing and increased blood pressure. Secondary smoke and even chewing tobacco can increase blood pressure.

Alcohol—blood pressure can be affected by having just one (women) or two (men) drinks a day.

Stress—your blood pressure can be temporarily elevated by stress.

2. Derail diabetes

While diabetes is treatable there is no getting away from the fact that it increases your risk of heart disease and stroke. It is also one of the modifiable risk factors for dementia.

Undiagnosed diabetes is common. In fact, the rule of halves also applies to diabetes, which means that half of the people living with diabetes are undiagnosed. Of those who have been diagnosed, only half receive appropriate treatment from a qualified health-care professional, and of those only half achieve their treatment targets. Furthermore, of this already small subset only half will live a life free from diabetes-related complications.

It doesn't have to be this way. Governments and health-care professionals have a lot of work to do to improve awareness, diagnosis, and outcomes. But you also have a personal responsibility and you owe it to yourself to take action to reduce your risk of diabetes or improve your outcomes if you have already been diagnosed with diabetes. As a first step, if you think you may be at risk why not make an appointment to speak to your doctor about having your urine or blood tested for sugar?

Guidelines vary from country to country, but diabetes screening has been recommended for anyone with a BMI over 25 who also have additional risk factors for diabetes (such as a sedentary lifestyle, high blood pressure, high cholesterol, a close relative with diabetes, history of diabetes in pregnancy). Blood-sugar testing has been recommended for anyone over the age of forty-five. If results from initial screening are normal, have a routine check every three years. Talk to your doctor about testing, which can take the form of a fasting blood-sugar test or a blood-sugar test taken at a random time.

Most cases of type 2 diabetes are preventable and some can even be reversed.

Modifiable risk factors that increase your risk of developing type 2 diabetes:

Being overweight or obese—the more fatty tissue you have, the more resistant your cells become to insulin.

High blood pressure—this increases your risk of type 2 diabetes.

Physical inactivity—being active uses up glucose for energy and makes your cells more sensitive to insulin. The more sedentary you are the greater your risk for diabetes.

Abnormal cholesterol and triglyceride levels—your risk of type 2 diabetes increases the lower your HDL. Having high triglyceride levels also increases your risk of type 2 diabetes.

Whether you are trying to prevent or control the disease you need to be careful about your food choices, weight, and activity levels. Becoming more physically active (see Chapter 7), following a Mediterranean diet (see Tip 3, below), and attaining and maintaining a healthy weight (see Tip 10) can help.

3. Shop for your brain

Eating a balanced diet is key to heart health. Know what you are eating, try to eat fresh food and cook from scratch. If you must eat processed or prepackaged food, read the labels and choose carefully.

Instead of going to the shop with a list of all the macro- and micro-nutrients that your brain requires, you could take a big-picture approach and keep your brain and heart in good shape by adopting a Mediterranean-style diet. People who follow a Mediterranean diet are less likely to develop heart disease and have a reduced risk of cognitive decline and Alzheimer's disease.

The Mediterranean diet emphasizes foods that are rich in omega-3 fatty acids, including whole grains, fresh fruits and vegetables, fish, and garlic. Long-term consumption of trans fats may compromise your health. Following the Mediterranean diet also means taking olive oil as a main source of fat. The Mediterranean diet has a healthier balance between omega-3 and omega-6 fatty acids than other Western diets, and it is important to have the proper ratio of these fatty acids in your diet. Omega-3 fatty acids help reduce inflammation, and most omega-6 fatty acids tend to promote inflammation. Both of these essential fatty acids, which are linked to preventing degenerative brain conditions, must come from your diet as your body can't make them.

Your brain enjoys nothing more than breathing in plenty of oxygen as you exercise, but to redeem the benefits of all that movement you need a good supply of iron running through your veins. This means topping up on foods such as green leafy vegetables like spinach, fortified cereal, dried fruit, and legumes.

Remember, studies have not identified individual nutrients as outstanding soloist performers in brain health. It is better to tap to the beat of an orchestra of nutrients from a medley of food types obtained from a balanced diet.

4. Control your cholesterol

One of the best ways to avoid cardiovascular disease is to keep your cholesterol at a healthy level. Knowing your cholesterol is crucial to understanding your risk for heart disease. Ask your doctor to do a cholesterol test, especially if a close relative has high cholesterol, heart disease, or has had a stroke. Abnormal cholesterol is often associated with high blood pressure and is related to similar life choices such as physical inactivity, being overweight, drinking too much alcohol, and consuming a lot of sugary foods.

High cholesterol affects people of all ages but making small changes can make a big difference. Sometimes the balance of cholesterol in your body goes awry as a consequence of an inherited problem, but often it is a consequence of eating too much animal fat or too many fatty foods, which is entirely under your control.

A simple blood test is used to measure total cholesterol, low- and high-density lipoproteins (LDL and HDL) and triglycerides. LDL transports cholesterol particles throughout your body via your blood. If LDL builds up on the walls of your arteries they can become hard and narrow, increasing your risk for heart disease. Lower LDL numbers are better for your health.

HDL picks up excess cholesterol and takes it out of your blood and back to your liver, thereby preventing build-up in your arteries. Higher HDL numbers are healthier.

Your blood will also contain triglycerides, a form of fat in your blood. Any calories that you eat but don't use immediately are converted to triglycerides and stored in fat cells.

Modifiable risk factors that increase your risk of high cholesterol are:

Poor diet—saturated fat, trans fats, red meat, and full-fat dairy increase cholesterol.

Obesity—a BMI of 30 or more.

Large waist—male 102cm/40in: female 89cm/35in.

Physical inactivity—exercise boosts HDL and makes LDL less harmful.

Smoking—the damage that smoking causes to your blood vessels increases the likelihood that fatty deposits will build up—smoking may also lower HDL.

Diabetes—high blood sugar damages the lining of your arteries and can lead to higher LDL and lower HDL.

5. Skip the salt

Sodium is an essential mineral. It helps to send nerve impulses and it also controls the fluid balance in your body. However, when there is too much sodium in your bloodstream it pulls water into your blood vessels, increasing the total amount of blood inside the vessels, placing a strain on your heart and increasing blood pressure. In some people excess sodium may lead to hypertension. Having less sodium in your diet may help to prevent or lower high blood pressure.

You can make changes gradually. Don't add salt to your food today. If you miss the seasoning, use black pepper, spices, or lemon instead. Avoid processed foods and takeout, which can be high in added salt. Why not try one day a week free from processed foods. When you go shopping, read the food labels and pay particular attention to the sodium content.

6. Hydrate

Make sure that you consume enough fluids every day so that your brain is kept hydrated and properly serviced with the energy and nutrients it needs to function well. Remember, you need water to remove toxins from your brain, too. We're often told to drink eight glasses of water per day, but that is overly simplistic. A better rule of thumb is to divide your weight in pounds by two and aim for that many ounces of water each day.

Drink fluids before, during, and after exercise. Make sure you adjust your intake to take account of hot weather. An increase in the frequency of urination or any other change in your usual pattern may signify an infection. Don't be tempted to reduce your fluid intake to lower urinary frequency or urgency, as this may lead to dehydration, especially if you have a kidney or urinary tract infection. Make an appointment to visit your doctor instead and follow their medical advice.

7. Watch what you drink

Choose your fluids wisely. You might also want to avoid drinking tea with meals as it prevents the uptake of iron. Avoid fluids that contain added sugar or caffeine.

Go easy on the alcohol, too. Heavy drinking is harmful to brain health. Bear in mind that excessive drinking can increase your blood pressure, harm your heart, and may even lead to stroke and brain damage. Drinking alcohol will also affect your weight and impair your sleep.

There is some evidence that a small amount of red wine can be beneficial. However, findings from a study that measured people's weekly alcohol intake, cognitive performance, and brain structure over thirty years found no protective effects of light drinking over total abstinence. While we had been aware that heavy drinking is harmful to brain health, this recent study revealed that even moderate drinking could impact negatively on the structure of the brain.

The study revealed a dose-dependent relationship between atrophy of the hippocampus and alcohol consumption. This means that the more you drink the greater the atrophy. Those who consume more than thirty units of alcohol per week have the highest risk of hippocampal wasting compared to non-drinkers. Even moderate drinkers (14–21 units per week) are three times more likely to have atrophy in their hippocampus than non-drinkers.

Guidelines vary from country to country and most don't take account of this recent research. Currently the guidelines are 14 units spread over a week.

Drinking any amount of alcohol increases the risk of damage to your health and as such there is no "safe" amount of alcohol. Government guidelines are for "low risk" rather than "no risk" consumption. To keep risks low it is safest not to drink more than 14 units of alcohol per week on a regular basis.

It's not just the number of units that matters either, the pattern of consumption is also important. If you do drink 14 units on a regular basis it should be spread over three or more days. Binge-drinking brings with it additional health risks. Just one or two heavy drinking days per week increase your risk. You should aim for several alcohol-free days each week.

Drinking at home can be problematic for health because we tend to pour larger measures. Invest in a proper measure and use it at home when you pour your own drinks so that you can keep an accurate eye on your alcohol consumption. A standard unit of alcohol is a half a pint of normal beer, a pub measure of spirits, a small glass of wine or of any other alcoholic drink. While meeting friends is great for brain health, if that involves going to the pub, consider alternating each alcoholic drink with a glass of water when socializing.

Drinking alcohol when the brain is still developing during adolescence and young adulthood may impair the growth of certain brain structures and can impair brain performance, including memory function. Consuming alcohol during adolescence, when a lot of us in Western society first begin drinking, can alter brain blood flow and electrical activity. Everyone is different, of course, and not all of us are equally sensitive to alcohol in our teens and early twenties, and other factors may influence the extent to which drinking alcohol affects brain development and functioning

8. Manage stress and stay connected

The relationship between stress, stroke, and heart disease is complex and not yet fully understood. It is possible that persistently elevated levels of stress hormones damage arteries and lead to high blood pressure, or it could be that poorly managed chronic stress leads to behaviors that make other risk factors worse. If you are chronically stressed you may exercise less, eat more, smoke or drink too much caffeine or alcohol. See Chapter 4 for practical tips to manage stress.

Loneliness experienced over long periods can act as a chronic stressor. Loneliness is a risk factor for heart disease and this may be because we try to cope with loneliness by drinking, smoking, or overeating. Loneliness is also associated with poor sleep and high blood pressure. In terms of heart health, staying connected with friends may be more important than physical exercise, smoking, or alcohol consumption because loneliness is a bigger cardiovascular risk factor than the other three.

9. Quit smoking

If you smoke, stop. Smokers have less oxygen flow to their brains and smoking is a major risk factor for heart disease. One in every two smokers will die of smoking-related disease and smokers are twice as likely to have a heart attack as non-smokers. As an ex-smoker I understand that quitting can be challenging. I went for the cold turkey approach and just stopped smoking one day, more than twenty years ago.

The key to my success was not to fall into the trap of talking about how much I missed the cigarettes or how tough I was finding it. I just told my brain from day one that I was a non-smoker and only allowed myself to say negative things about smoking. My brain was very obedient and within about three to four weeks I couldn't even bear the smell of someone else's cigarette, let alone contemplate lighting one.

It may help to learn more about why you smoke or you may need support to help you through the process. It does help to know that cravings only last a few minutes at a time, so when you crave a cigarette take deep breaths in through your nose and out through your mouth, drink a glass of water, brush your teeth, deploy a distraction and you will find that after three or four minutes the urge will pass.

Everyone is different, of course, and what worked for me isn't necessarily going to work for you. Cutting down gradually might work better for you than sudden cessation. You could start by smoking one fewer cigarette today. Or maybe you could try stubbing out at least one cigarette halfway through today. Or tomorrow delay lighting your first cigarette by ten minutes. Try that for a few mornings then challenge yourself to delay the first one by fifteen minutes and so on. Another approach is to try reducing your daily cigarette intake by 10 percent so that over time you eventually quit.

If you are currently a smoker, quitting smoking is the single best thing that you can do for your heart health. It's never too late to quit smoking. Within hours of quitting smoking your blood pressure and heart rate return to normal and the carbon monoxide levels in your blood drop to normal. Within one day your risk of heart attack begins to fall.

One year after quitting your risk of coronary heart disease is about half that of a smoker. Fifteen years after quitting your risk for coronary heart disease returns to the level of a non-smoker. Your risk of stroke returns to the same level as a non-smoker between five and fifteen years after quitting. If you have already had a heart attack, giving up smoking halves your risk of another attack.

When it comes to smoking it is never too late to stop. No matter what age you are you will benefit from quitting. The cortex in the brains of former smokers increases each year that we stay smoke free. The brain has the capacity to repair itself, provided you quit—and the only person who can do that is you. Make a plan and pledge to quit today. Google "how to quit smoking" and find a method that suits you.

10. Attain and maintain a healthy weight

Being overweight or obese increases your risk of developing high blood pressure and heart disease and as a consequence is not good for brain health. Being underweight is not healthy either. The key is to identify your ideal weight, attain it and maintain it.

Small changes can make big differences. Even something simple like changing the color or size of your plate can reduce the amount of food you consume at one sitting. If you want to eat less, select a plate that has a high color contrast with what you plan to serve for dinner. When there is a low contrast between food color and plate color people tend to serve themselves portions that are 30 percent larger than when there is a high contrast. So if you want to eat more green vegetables serve them on a green plate. Have a snack-free day or a sugar-free day each week. Or try reducing your portions by 10 percent. Try cooking your meals from scratch using only fresh ingredients. Aim to spend longer preparing your food than you do eating it.

You know from Chapter 3 that when you are sleep deprived you are less able to resist temptation and you are likely to experience increased hunger and appetite due to elevated levels of endocannabinoids. You are also likely to consume more between meals and more likely to eat unhealthy snacks between meals. If you are serious about losing weight you will also need to make sure that you are getting enough sleep.

Getting physically active will help with weight loss, plus it's good for your brain and your heart. Exercising doesn't just burn calories it also strengthens connections in your brain in a way that gives you greater control over your impulses and emotions—including your impulse to eat. Get active to resist the temptation to eat junk. The next chapter explains more about how physical activity benefits brain health.

HEART—PART TWO

Goals—Action Plan—Personal Profile

Set your goals, devise your action plan, and create your personal profile for Heart.

Brain Health Goals: Heart

Answering the following questions, using information from your Food Log, medical tests, and Assessments so far, will help you to set heart-healthy goals to boost your brain health.

The more risk factors you have the greater your chance of developing cardiovascular disease, which in turn impacts on the health of your brain. If your assessment reveals multiple risk factors I would strongly recommend working with a medical professional to minimize your risk and, where relevant, devise a treatment plan to bring risk factors under control.

Guidelines vary but it has been recommended that all adults aged over twenty should have their risk for stroke and other cardiovascular diseases checked every four to six years, then work with their doctor to determine risk and treatment.

Q1. Blood pressure

Blood pressure (BP) is measured using two numbers: Systolic/Diastolic. Generally speaking:

Optimal BP = between 90/60 mm Hg and 12/80 mm Hg

High BP = 140/90 mm Hg or higher

At risk for high BP = between 120/80 mm Hg and 140/90 mm Hg

Low BP = 90/60 mm Hg or lower

My blood pressure is ___/__

I don't know my blood pressure ☐

Heart Goal No. 1a

Get my blood pressure tested regularly ☐

I have healthy blood pressure ☐
I am at risk of developing high blood pressure ☐
I have high blood pressure ☐
I have high blood pressure and follow my doctor's advice
    to keep it under control ☐
I have multiple modifiable risk factors for high blood pressure ☐
I have low blood pressure ☐

Heart Goal No. 1b

I want to take action to reduce my blood pressure ☐

No action required: I have healthy blood pressure and I get it
tested regularly ☐

Q2. Cholesterol

Your health-care professional will help you to interpret your scores. Your doctor will set a target for you based on your personal overall risk factors. As a general guide, for healthy adults total cholesterol levels should be 5 mmol/L or less. Your LDL level should be 3 mmol/L or lower. Your HDL level should be above 1 mmol/L. The ratio of total cholesterol to HDL (calculate by dividing total by HDL) should be below 4. Your triglyceride level should be less than 1.7 mmol/L.

Note: Guidelines and measurement mode (milligrams or millimoles) differ across countries. I've used UK/European here.

My cholesterol/HDL ratio is ___
I don't know my cholesterol levels ☐

Heart Goal No. 2a

Get my cholesterol tested ☐

I have healthy cholesterol levels ☐
I have unhealthy cholesterol levels ☐
I have multiple modifiable risk factors for cholesterol ☐

Heart Goal No. 2b

I want to take action to get my cholesterol within the healthy range ☐

No action required: I have healthy cholesterol levels and I get it tested regularly ☐

Q3. Diabetes and blood sugar

I don't know my blood sugar levels ☐
I don't know whether I have diabetes or pre-diabetes ☐

Heart Goal No. 3a

I will ask my doctor about whether I need blood sugar or diabetes tests ☐

I have healthy blood sugar levels ☐
I don't have pre-diabetes ☐
I don't have diabetes ☐
I have unhealthy blood sugar levels ☐
I have pre-diabetes ☐
I have diabetes ☐
I have multiple risk factors for diabetes ☐

Heart Goal No. 3b

I want to get my blood sugar within the healthy range ☐

I want to reduce my risk for diabetes ☐

I would like to control my diabetes better ☐

No action required: I have no risk factors, I have healthy blood sugar levels, and I don't have diabetes or pre-diabetes ☐

Q4. Weight

a) Body Mass Index (BMI)

BMI =____

Obese = BMI of 30.0 and above. Overweight = BMI 25 to 29.9.

Healthy = BMI 18.5 to 24.9. Underweight = BMI less than 18.5

Waist measurement_____

Regardless of your height or build your health is at risk if you have a waist measurement of greater than 94 cm/37 in for men or 80 cm/31.5 in for women.

My weight is within the healthy range for my height ☐
My weight is either above or below the healthy range for my height ☐
My BMI is within the healthy range ☐
My BMI is either above or below the healthy range ☐
My waist circumference is within the healthy range ☐
My waist circumference is not within the healthy range ☐

Heart Goal No. 4a

I want to get my weight ☐   BMI ☐   waist ☐   within the healthy range

No action required: my weight, BMI, and waist are within the healthy range ☐

---

b) Base your answer on your *Assessment: Food Log*, government portion guidelines, and the food pyramid.

I have a healthy balanced diet ☐
I consume too many calories ☐
I consume too few calories ☐
I consume unhealthy amounts of salt ☐
I consume unhealthy amounts of sugar ☐
I consume unhealthy amounts of fat ☐
I don't consume enough water ☐

Heart Goal No. 4b

I want to modify my diet to reduce my risk of cardiovascular disease ☐

No action required: I eat a balanced heart-healthy diet ☐

Q5. Smoking

I am a smoker Yes ☐   No ☐

Heart Goal No. 5

I want to quit smoking ☐

No action required: I don't smoke ☐

Q6. Alcohol

My alcohol consumption is greater than government guidelines ☐

Heart Goal No. 6

I want to reduce my alcohol intake ☐

I want to change the pattern of my drinking ☐

No action required: I'm happy with my alcohol intake and pattern of drinking ☐

No action required: I don't drink alcohol ☐

Completing the table below using the information from your Heart Goals will help you to characterize your current healthy habits and prioritize any heart habits that need fixing. Tick the box that applies then enter any items that need fixing into the Brain Health Action Plan on the next page.

	Healthy	Needs fixing	Priority*
Blood pressure			
Cholesterol levels			
Blood sugar			
Diabetes			
Weight			
BMI			
Diet			
Smoking			
Alcohol consumption			
Salt intake			
Sugar intake			
Fat intake			
Other			

*High, medium, or low

Physical activity, critical for both heart and brain health, is covered in detail in the next chapter.

Brain Health Action Plan: Heart

Enter your heart habits that need fixing into the Brain Health Action column in the table opposite. Indicate whether the action is attainable with relative ease in the short term (quick fix) or will require more time and effort to achieve (long term). The ten tips that you have just read should help you to break each action into practical steps. Prioritize the actions in the order you would like to work on them (1 = tackle first). *You will find a completed sample in the back of the book.*

Brain Health Action	Order	Steps	Quick fix	Long term

Personal Profile: Heart

Using your scores in the **Brain Health Goals: Heart** section as a guide, complete this table. Indicate whether your scores are healthy, borderline, or unhealthy. From that you can determine whether your current pattern of behavior is a brain-healthy asset or a risk that could compromise your brain health and make you vulnerable to dementia in later life. Finally, indicate the aspects that you would like to fix, improve, or maintain and prioritize them for inclusion in your Brain Health Plan in Chapter 9.

Aspect	Healthy	Borderline	Unhealthy	Asset	Risk	Maintain	Improve	Fix	Priority
Blood pressure									
Cholesterol									
Weight/BMI/Diet									
Diabetes/ Blood sugar									
Smoking									
Alcohol									
Total									

100 Days to a Younger Brain

PROGRAM DAYS 17–23: LOVING YOUR HEART

You should now have a clearer understanding of your cardiovascular risk factors, your personal goals, and the actions that you need to take to protect your heart to benefit your brain health. You will combine your heart profile with the other profiles that you will create as you complete the program to build your overall Brain Health Profile in Chapter 9. You will also select at least one of your heart actions to add to your overall Brain Health Plan.

100-DAY DIARY

You can record the steps that you are taking toward your program goals in the 100-Day Diary at the back of the book. For example:

- I made an appointment to get my blood pressure checked.
- I read the labels in the supermarket and avoided items with added sugar.
- I skipped wine with dinner.
- I cooked my dinner from scratch with fresh ingredients.

You can also celebrate your healthy habits by recording them in your 100-Day Diary.

7

Get Physical

*"Lack of activity destroys the good condition of every
human being, while movement and methodical
physical exercise save it and preserve it."*
Plato

PHYSICAL—PART ONE

As children we run and jump for the sheer joy of it. As teens many of us play sports but ditch the activity relatively early in adulthood to become sofa-sitting or sideline spectators. Some people are fortunate to have jobs that offer opportunities for aerobic and anaerobic activity, but millions of us sit at desks all day accruing the negative impact of inactivity. By middle age, while a scattering of us consciously seek ways to take exercise for the health benefits, many of us lead increasingly sedentary lives.

Did you know that the more steps (literally) you take to get fitter, the healthier your brain becomes? There is no magic pill you can pop to improve your memory but regularly stepping out for a hike or even a brisk walk can nourish your brain. Dancing, gardening, and housework will give your brain a boost, too. Physical activity has direct benefits on the structure and functioning of your brain. In contrast, living a sedentary life of physical inactivity increases risk for heart disease and dementia.

The innovative tips in this chapter will get you moving to benefit brain health, and keeping the Physical Log and completing the assessments will give you great insights into your physical activity levels, which will help you to transform your physical fitness and boost your brain health. You will use this information to create your personal physical profile, set goals, and devise a physical action plan in Part Two of this chapter. First let's look to neuroscience to help us to understand why physical activity is a real boon for brain health and why we all need to sit less.

Quick Question: Physical

Thinking about your usual pattern (don't count time spent asleep)

How much time do you spend sitting or lying down on a typical work day? _____

How much time do you spend sitting or lying down on a typical day off? _____

Brain Gains: What Has Physical Activity Got to Do with Brain Health?

Having billions of neurons means that your brain is the most energy-demanding organ in your body. *Your brain only weighs about 2 percent of your body but uses 20–25 percent of your body energy every day just to keep your brain working*. Based on the Brazilian brain soup count, it costs six calories to run one billion neurons, that's 516 calories out of your 2000-calorie daily entitlement just to keep your 86 billion neurons ticking over. Your brain consumes a lot of oxygen and nutrients and needs to be constantly informed of your body's needs and available resources. It depends on its vast neuronal networks to provide that information. Your ability to learn, think, and remember is closely linked to your glucose levels and the ability of your brain to efficiently use this energy source. You know from reading the previous chapter that your brain health is very much linked to heart health and to the health and integrity of the blood vessels that carry the oxygen and nutrients around your body and your brain.

Your brain needs oxygen to thrive and cannot survive for more than a few minutes without it. This is one of the reasons why exercise is critical for brain health.

When you start exercising, the blood flowing to your brain carries extra oxygen and nutrients to your neurons. It seems your brain is poised to take advantage of this and we think that the increase in oxygen may help to stimulate the production of new nerve cells.

Physical activity refers to any bodily movement that requires you to expend energy. This includes the movements that you make as you go about your daily life at home, at work, and at leisure. Physical activity also includes physical exercise—a subset that is structured, repetitive, and planned. In contrast to the general nature of physical activity, exercise usually has a purpose related to some aspect of physical fitness.

Assessment: Physical Log

On Days 24–30, keep a **Physical Log**. Record how much time you spend in each type of activity while at work, commuting to work (transport), at home, during leisure time, and how long you spent sitting. You will use this detail (work, transport, home, and leisure) to complete the International Physical Activity Questionnaire (IPAQ) later in the chapter. If you have a wrist tracker or any other type of app that records your activity levels you can use this to help you to complete the log and the questionnaire below. **DO NOT** record bouts of activity of less than ten minutes duration.

Duration: Record all activity in minutes.

Moderate activity: With moderate activity you will be active at a comfortable pace. You will still be able to carry on a conversation but your heart rate and breathing will increase. You will also feel warm or sweat slightly. Examples of moderate aerobic exercise are: brisk walking (15 minutes per mile), cycling (less than 10 miles per hour), ballroom dancing, medium-paced swimming, gardening, and doubles tennis.

Vigorous activity: You will no longer be able to carry on a conversation and you will be concentrating hard on the activity. You will be breathing heavily, have a fast heart rate, and be sweating. Examples include: jogging, running, circuit training, heavy gardening, dancing (hip hop, salsa, street), and active sports (soccer, squash, aerobics, singles tennis).

Total minutes = Mon + Tues + Weds + Thurs + Fri + Sat + Sun

Total weekday minutes sitting = Total minutes minus your "weekend" days or days off

MET minutes per week represent the amount of energy you use carrying out physical activity each week.

- One MET is the amount of energy that you use when you are at rest.
- Walking = 3.3 METs (i.e., when you walk you use 3.3 times the amount of energy you use when you are at rest)
- Moderate activity = 4 METs
- Vigorous activity = 8 METs

Record physical activity duration in minutes. Only record physical activity that you did for at least ten minutes at a time.

You will find a completed sample in the back of the book.

Type	Life domain	Mon Mins	Tues Mins	Weds Mins	Thurs Mins	Fri Mins	Sat Mins	Sun Mins	Days*	Total Mins	MET minutes
Vigorous	Work										Vigorous total mins (work + leisure) x 8
	Leisure										
											Vigorous MET minutes = ___
Moderate	Work										Moderate total mins (work + home + leisure) x 4
	Home										
	Leisure										Moderate MET minutes = ___
Walking	Work										Walking total mins (work + transport + leisure) x 3.3
	Transport										
	Leisure										Walking MET minutes = ___
Total MET minutes											Vigorous + Moderate + Walking =___
Sitting minutes											Weekdays sitting total
	Work										
	Other										

*Number of days on which you engage in the activity.

When you have logged your physical activity for a week, use the information to complete the International Physical Activity Questionnaire. **Assessment: IPAQ** below.

Use the information in this log to inform your answers to Questions 2 and 3 in Part Two of this chapter (Brain Health Goals: Physical).

Assessment: IPAQ

The IPAQ questions ask about the seven days of the **Physical Log** that you completed this week. Answer each question even if you do not consider yourself to be an active person.

1. On how many days did you do vigorous physical activities?

   Number of days ____

Skip to Question 3 if you recorded no vigorous activity.

2. How much time did you usually spend on one of those days doing vigorous physical activities?

   Number of minutes per day ___

3. On how many days did you do moderate physical activities? Please do not include walking.

   Number of days ____

Skip to Question 5 if you recorded no moderate activity.

4. How much time did you usually spend on one of those days doing moderate physical activities?

   Number of minutes per day ___

5. On how many days did you walk for at least ten minutes at a time?

   Number of days per week ___

Skip to Question 7 if you recorded no walking activity.

6. How much time did you usually spend walking on one of those days?

   Number of minutes per day ___

7. How much time did you spend sitting on a weekday?

   Number of minutes per weekday ___

What your IPAQ scores mean

To calculate whether your physical activity can be classified as high, moderate, or low, you need to take account of both the total volume of your physical activity (MET minutes) and the number of days that you take part in the activity.*

Vigorous Activity Days (IPAQ Que. 1) _____
Vigorous MET minutes (Physical Log) _____
Moderate Activity Days (IPAQ Que. 3) _____
Moderate MET minutes (Physical Log) _____
Walking Days (IPAQ Que. 5) _____
Walking MET minutes (Physical Log) _____

Follow the instructions below to determine your activity levels. *You will find a completed sample in the back of the book.*

High levels of activity

The two criteria for classification as "high" are:

- vigorous-intensity activity on at least three days achieving a minimum total physical activity of at least 1,500 MET minutes/ week

OR

- seven or more days of any combination of walking, moderate-intensity, or vigorous-intensity activities, achieving a minimum total physical activity of at least 3,000 MET minutes/week.

---

* Where walking, moderate, and vigorous activity time exceeds 180 minutes for any one day the score recorded needs to be capped at 180 minutes. This would give a maximum of 21 hours of activity per week for each category (3 hours x 7 days).

To meet the criteria to be classified as engaging in high levels of physical activity you must engage in a combination of walking, moderate-intensity, and/or vigorous-intensity activity on at least seven days a week.

If you recorded four days of moderate-intensity and three days of walking you would have achieved at least seven days.

Similarly if you reported three days of vigorous-intensity, three days of moderate-intensity and three days walking, you would also be classified as having achieved at least seven days.

Moderate levels of activity

Engaging in the equivalent of thirty minutes of at least moderate-intensity activity on most days is categorized as moderate.

The pattern of activity to be classified as "moderate" is either of the following criteria:

- three or more days of vigorous-intensity activity of at least twenty minutes per day

OR

- five or more days of moderate-intensity activity and/or walking of at least thirty minutes per day

OR

- five or more days of any combination of walking, moderate-intensity, or vigorous-intensity activities, achieving a minimum total physical activity of at least 600 MET minutes/week.

Meeting at least one of the above criteria would be defined as accumulating a minimum level of activity and therefore be classified as "moderate."

To be classified as "moderately active" you need to undertake activity on at least five days a week.

If you report two days of moderate-intensity and three days of walking, that would count as at least five days. Similarly, if you report two days of vigorous-intensity, two days of moderate-intensity, and two days of walking it would also count as at least five days per week.

Low levels of activity

Scores that don't meet the criteria for moderate- or high-intensity activity are considered to be low physical activity level.

Level of activity score High ☐ Moderate ☐ Low ☐

Use your IPAQ scores to answer Question 1, Part Two in this chapter (Brain Health Goals: Physical).

Health recommendations

You will be familiar with public health recommendations for physical activity of thirty minutes of moderate intensity five times per week. It is important to point out that these recommendations are based on leisure-time physical activity. By completing the **Assessment: IPAQ** you will understand that accumulating just thirty minutes of moderate-intensity activity across all of your life domains on five days a week would be incredibly low. Essentially, that would be equivalent to the background or base levels of activity that most adults would accumulate on any day. To attain health benefits when measuring physical activity across all domains a higher cut-point is needed.

Greater health benefits are associated with higher levels of activity. There is no public health agreement on the exact amounts needed for maximal benefit but IPAQ calculations are based on counting at least one hour per day or more of at least moderate-intensity activity above the base level of physical activity. If you take 5,000 steps per day as a base level of activity, completing 12,500 steps per day or the equivalent in moderate and vigorous activities is considered a high-level activity.

Physical exercise is good for brain health because it helps to maintain the blood flow and the supply of oxygen and nutrients to the brain. It also reduces risk of cardiovascular disease and cerebrovascular[28] events such as stroke. Physical activity has a positive impact on cardiovascular and dementia risk factors, including high blood pressure, obesity, and type 2 diabetes. Physical activity helps to reduce the brain's exposure to neurotoxins including beta-amyloid, a build-up of which is implicated in Alzheimer's disease.

Brain changing

Physical activity literally changes your brain. It seems to enhance the connections in your brain by stimulating the release of brain fertilizer (BDNF). It also supports your brain cells and helps new ones to grow, which goes some way toward explaining why your brain shrinks less as you age if you remain physically active. Exercising also makes your brain more plastic. This means that areas of your brain (such as the hippocampus and prefrontal cortex) are able to rise to the challenge of learning and you will see improvements in memory, attention, and the speed with which you can process information.

Exercise also helps the connections between neurons in your brain to work better. When the emotional center in your brain (amygdala) and your executive control center (prefrontal cortex) have strong connections it becomes easier for you to maintain a healthy weight. This is because this stronger connectivity gives you greater control over your impulses and your emotions, including your impulse to eat. Of course, exercise will also keep your weight on track because it burns fat, too.

Fringe benefits

While physical exercise is fundamental to physical health, other fringe benefits associated with such exercise include the release of "feel-good" chemicals in the brain called endorphins. These endorphins improve mood and reduce symptoms of depression, stress, and anxiety. Physical activity can also buffer against some of the negative impacts that chronic stress can have on the brain through the reduction of cortisol levels.

Maintaining physical fitness can also help you to remain independent as you age and will give you more energy to do the things that you want to do, not less. Being active means that you will sleep more soundly too, and sleep is something your brain thrives on. People who walk more are less likely to be lonely and more likely to be socially active.

Exercise, memory, and dementia

Have you ever bought a gym membership you've rarely (or never) used? Or perhaps you've made a New Year's resolution to get physically fit only to find yourself flopped in front of the TV or your laptop every night by 1 February. You might be a little less shy of the treadmill if you knew that exercise tones your brain as well as your butt, reducing your risk of dementia in the process.

When compared to people who lead sedentary lives, it's not just people who engage in high levels of physical exercise that reduce their risk of cognitive decline, engaging in low to moderate levels of physical activity also appears to be beneficial. People in their late fifties and early sixties who report being physically active demonstrate better general cognitive function, episodic memory, processing speed, and executive control than those who don't.

Most studies looking at the impact of physical exercise on memory and other cognitive functions are usually carried out on adults over the age of fifty-five. But one study that investigated younger adults over a seventeen-year period found that physical exercise at the age of thirty-six was associated with slower memory decline between the ages of forty-three and fifty-three. People who had been engaging in physical exercise at the age of thirty-six and at the age of forty-three had the lowest decay in memory at fifty-three. People who stopped exercising at thirty-six had less protection against memory decline than those who started exercising at thirty-six.

Generally speaking, people who are physically active throughout life have better cognitive function in later life and so maintain this for longer. But it also seems that benefits can be gained by taking up or resuming physical activity as we get older.

No-Brainer: Get physically active.

Brain Drains: What Happens in Your Brain Without Physical Activity?

While following daily exercise recommendations is good for your heart and your brain, it's not the whole story because physical inactivity and a sedentary lifestyle represent health hazards in and of themselves. Exercising for thirty minutes a day is great but what you do for the rest of the day matters, too. Do you jog in the morning then sit in front of a computer all day without moving, or do you go to the gym after work for an hour then flop in front of a TV for the rest of the evening?

Physical inactivity

Meeting the recommended physical activity guidelines is not enough. You also need to consider how much time you spend being physically inactive, because too long spent in sedentary behavior increases your risk for chronic diseases.

While physical activity has a direct benefit on your brain's structure and function, physical inactivity is associated with a number of cardiovascular risk factors, including diabetes and high blood pressure, which in turn are associated with increased risk of dementia. Physical inactivity is also associated with depression. In fact, about four million cases of Alzheimer's disease around the globe are potentially attributable to physical inactivity. As we age we tend to become less physically active and this disuse can lead to premature aging, heart disease, depression, and obesity.

Physical inactivity accelerates the aging process while physical activity slows it down. The choice is yours to make.

Sitting duck

In addition to becoming more physically active we also need to sit less. Our societal obsession with sitting is, quite frankly, a disaster for heart health. Prolonged periods of sitting slows your metabolism, affecting the body's ability to regulate blood pressure, blood sugar, and break down body fat. It's easy to see how a sedentary lifestyle is associated with increased risk of cardiovascular disease and type 2 diabetes. It's also linked to obesity and being overweight.

The adverse effects of sedentary behavior apply even if you meet physical activity guidelines. I'll repeat that even if you are getting your 150 minutes of exercise a week, sitting too much comes with its own risks for your heart. Physical inactivity is one of the seven modifiable risk factors for dementia and the fourth leading cause of death in the world.

On average, in addition to time spent sleeping, we spend seven hours every day sitting or lying. How do you compare? We spend the bulk of our days on our butts at a computer, at a desk, watching TV, at the wheel of our car, or on a bus, tram, or train. Working from home may make matters worse. Patterns of sedentary behavior established in childhood persist with age, so in addition to changing our own habits it's really important to get our kids and grandkids moving more and sitting less.

Adults who report more than four hours a day of screen time are at greater risk of heart attack when compared to adults who log less than two hours a day in front of the TV or other screen-based entertainment. Obese people sit for two hours and fifteen minutes per day more than lean people. Slimmer people in the past actually ate more than we do today but they burned more energy because they were on their feet more.

It's not rocket science. You burn on average one calorie per minute sitting, two per minute standing and four per minute walking.

Older adults spend between eight and a half hours and ten hours sitting or lying every day. Social norms that tell us to slow down as we age are not helpful. Aging by itself is not the problem, we experience worse decline due to our lack of physical fitness and sedentary life choices. Moving more and sitting less will help to ensure that you experience the most beneficial rate of physical decline possible in later life. As you get older you need to do less sitting, not more.

When we park ourselves in one spot for hours on end the lack of movement reduces the flow of blood and the amount of oxygen entering your brain. As a consequence you may experience a drop in your ability to concentrate. If you slump at your desk with inward drooping shoulders, the hunched position of your body leaves little room for your lungs to expand. Your poor posture shrinks your chest cavity, temporarily limiting the amount of oxygen your lungs can take in.

When you sit for long periods of time you don't burn fat as well as you do when you keep moving because prolonged sitting temporarily deactivates the enzyme that breaks down fat. Sitting for hours at a time without standing can constrict the arteries in your legs, impeding blood flow. This can raise blood pressure and, over time, lead to heart disease, which negatively impacts on brain health.

No-Brainer: Sit less.

Summary

- Exercise is critical for brain health. It helps to maintain the blood flow and the supply of oxygen and nutrients to the brain and reduces risk for cardiovascular disease and stroke.
- Physical activity also helps to reduce the brain's exposure to neurotoxins including beta-amyloid, a build-up of which is implicated in Alzheimer's disease.
- Physical exercise gives rise to the growth of new neurons in the hippocampus and also helps the connections between neurons to work better.
- Physical inactivity is associated with a number of cardiovascular risk factors, including diabetes and high blood pressure, that in turn are associated with increased risk of dementia.
- Physical inactivity is also associated with depression.
- About four million cases of Alzheimer's disease around the globe are potentially attributable to physical inactivity.
- Physical inactivity accelerates the aging process while physical activity slows it down.
- Exercise and a healthy diet don't just allow you to live longer, they allow you to live better.
- Prolonged periods of sitting slow metabolism, affecting the body's ability to regulate blood pressure, blood sugar, and break down body fat.

Brain Changers: What You Can Do

Physical activity is fundamental to brain health. It would be foolish not to find ways to embrace it every day. Getting physically active reduces your risk of more than thirty chronic diseases, including heart disease and dementia. You'll not only live longer you'll live better. In addition it will boost your other brain-healthy habits because physical activity will help you to maintain a healthy weight, manage stress and mood, plus you'll sleep better.

There are 1,440 minutes in every day, so spend at least thirty of them doing some kind of physical activity. However, it's not just about being physically active for thirty minutes each day, you also need to change your sitting habits and move more throughout the day. The tips below offer some practical ways to actively invest in brain health.

TEN PRACTICAL TIPS TO GET PHYSICALLY ACTIVE

1. Exercise every day.
2. Safety first.
3. Sit less.
4. Stand more.
5. Straighten up.
6. Move more.
7. Swap some screen time for active hobbies.
8. Strength and balance.
9. Rest and recovery.
10. Play.

1. Exercise every day

Aim to exercise every day and don't let age get in the way. It really is an all-rounder: good for physical, mental, and brain health. Exercise can't be optional nor is it a luxury. It is one of the most important things you can do for your brain and your heart so you need to make it a part of your daily routine.

You need to do at least 150 minutes of moderate aerobic activity or seventy-five minutes of vigorous activity each week. Guidelines suggest splitting that over five days, which is good advice but I wouldn't see that as an excuse to vegetate two days a week. Do some form of physical activity every day.

If you already take regular exercise, well done—your heart and your brain are already benefiting. Why not try to increase your activity time by 10 percent or change your routine a bit and introduce some variety. If you've never exercised before, start small—why not try a fifteen-minute walk after dinner this evening?

Don't underestimate the benefits of walking. Regular walkers have longer and better-quality sleep. Walking is associated with sharper thinking, enhanced creativity, and improved mood. Walking can help boost cognitive function and rejuvenate your brain. Whatever your ability or mobility, you need to find a way to get physically active.

2. Safety first

Physical activity is generally safe for everyone, at any age. People who are physically fit have less chance of injury than those who are not fit. Always exercise safely and seek the advice of your doctor before taking on a new exercise regime if you:

- Are over fifty and are not used to energetic activity.
- Have a diagnosed chronic condition such as diabetes, heart disease, or osteoarthritis, or if you have symptoms such as chest pain or pressure, dizziness, or joint pain.

Match your level of effort to your level of fitness. If chronic illness, mobility issues, or a degenerative condition prevent you doing the recommended amount of physical activity, be as active as you are able to be. If you have mobility or health issues that make getting regular exercise challenging, be imaginative, do some research or ask members of your medical team for suggestions so that you can exercise safely within the constraints of your condition.

- Start slowly, and build your level of activity over time, particularly if you haven't been active for a long time.
- Learn about the types and amounts of activity that are right for you.
- Choose activities that are appropriate for you.
- Choose a safe place to do your activity.
- Use safety equipment, such as a helmet for bike riding and the correct shoes for walking or jogging.
- Be sure to drink plenty of fluids while you are exercising.

- Warm up your muscles and stretch before you exercise.
- If you feel faint or dizzy, have a pain, or feel in anyway unwell stop the activity immediately.

Just thirty minutes a day of physical exercise can reduce the risk of a heart attack. If you haven't been active for a while, start small—you can break your thirty minutes into two or three shorter sessions but make sure each session is at least ten minutes long. Find ways to incorporate exercise into your daily routine—walk to work or take the stairs.

3. Sit less

You need to break up long spells of sitting with bouts of moving for at least one to two minutes. If your job involves extended periods of sitting, get up and walk around at least every two hours if you are a younger adult and every hour if you are an older adult. When I'm working at my laptop for long periods, which is most days, I set an alarm for every thirty minutes to remind me to move for a couple of minutes. It's important to avoid long periods of sitting at work or at home in front of a screen. If you work at a desk, don't sit for some of your tasks. For example, you could open your post or take phone calls standing. If colleagues are allowed regular "smoking breaks" you could consider taking regular walking breaks to reduce your sitting time. Walk rather than sit during your tea or coffee break. After lunch, get up from the table and move about instead of spending your entire lunch break sitting.

Avoid long stints sitting in front of the TV, computer, or playing console games. If you are struggling to exercise for thirty minutes every day it's pretty crazy to spend more than an hour or two watching TV every evening. Life is precious and short. TV is great, don't get me wrong, I love a good box set myself, but it is a passive activity that encourages sedentary behavior. It's not about cutting it out altogether, it's about balance and making conscious decisions about how you use your precious time. Consider setting limits for yourself in advance. Take conscious note of how much time you are sitting without moving.

Get up and move around or go upstairs during the ad breaks or when you complete a level of a game. If you follow sport, try standing for some of the game while you watch it on TV. Make sure to move at least once every hour or every thirty minutes if you can manage it. Ditch the remote and change your channels old school. If you tend to binge-watch box sets for hours on end, force yourself to get up and walk around for a couple of minutes between each episode. You might find that this will help you to resist the temptation to watch the entire season in one night.

4. Stand more

Spend more time standing, but don't go overboard. Prolonged standing without opportunities to sit is not good either. The trick is to alternate between standing and sitting and avoid prolonged periods of either. Start to view standing as a form of exercise. *If you reduced your daily sitting time from eight hours to six hours by standing for two hours every day instead, the net effect is the equivalent of running six marathons a year.* Try to make a point of standing for specific activities like talking on the phone or on your commute to work. However, try not to stand in the same position for long periods and avoid wearing high heels if you do have to stand for prolonged periods.

Our brains actually perform better when we stand. In addition to being bad for your health, sitting for prolonged periods can lead to mental fatigue and lack of motion can push your body into sleep mode.

Standing desks are a fantastic invention, but you don't have to buy one, you can improvise by placing your laptop on a box on your desk. Consider taking meetings or holding conversations while standing. Sir Muir Gray, Oxford professor, physician, and public health adviser, who has been very vocal about the lethal dangers of sitting, stands for a quarter of his working day. He is very disciplined about it and makes sure that he stands for thirty minutes every two hours. I have tried this myself and it does take a lot of discipline and some advance planning. I'm still working on it.

5. Straighten up

Obviously you will still spend a significant portion of your day sitting, so it is important to minimize the impact of poor posture. When seated, try to keep your head straight, not tilted up or down or angled to the left or right. You may need to reposition your workstation to achieve this. Push your hips as far back in your chair as they will go and adjust your seat height so that your knees are slightly lower than your hips and your feet are flat on the floor.

You don't need to sit rigidly, it is possible to relax and have good posture. Try not to tuck your feet under the chair or cross your legs above your knees. Ideally your computer screen should be straight in front of you, about two or three inches above your seated eye level. If you are using a laptop you may need to place it on some large books or a box.

When you stand, keep your shoulders level and rolled back and use your stomach muscles to keep your body straight. Watch your posture when you are walking, too: heel to toe, using your muscles to hold your tummy and butt in line with the rest of your body. Avoid arching your back and looking down at your feet. Take in the world around you. Walking is a great opportunity to feed your senses and can be almost meditative.

If your physical activity regime includes running, try to keep your head looking forward, try not to bend at the waist, hunch your shoulders or lift your knees too high. Increasing the amount of time you spend standing and exercising will help you to sleep better but if your mattress is a bit tired consider investing in a new one with firm support.

6. Move more

We all lead such busy lives that sometimes it can seem like there simply aren't enough hours in the day. I understand that, and doing something like going to the gym every day can take out a chunk of time that you might feel you can't afford. Exercise is an investment in yourself. You need to tell yourself that you are worth it. Find ways to incorporate more movement into your daily routine.

- Get off the bus or train a couple of stops early.
- Park a little further away from your destination.
- Consider walking or cycling to work, if that's a realistic option.
- Take the stairs as much as possible.
- Walk while you are on the phone.
- Walk to talk to a colleague instead of emailing them.
- Meet friends for a walk rather than for a coffee.
- Housework counts as moderate exercise, so attack it with gusto.

7. Swap some screen time for active hobbies

Cut down on screen time and replace it with an active hobby like gardening, DIY, dancing, drumming, hiking, bird-watching, or juggling instead. It really doesn't matter what the hobby is once you enjoy it and it makes you feel good. Consider getting involved in community-based activities, join walking groups, attend dance classes, or volunteer for the local beach or park clean-up.

8. Strength and balance

Aerobic exercise is great for your heart and your brain but you also need to do strength and balance exercises at least two to three days a week. That means doing muscle-strengthening activities that work all major muscle groups (legs, hips, back abdomen, chest, shoulders, and arms).

Bone-strengthening activities include brisk walking, moderate-resistance weightlifting, stair climbing, carrying shopping, exercise bands, digging, heavy gardening, and cross-training machines.

Muscle-strengthening activities include weight machines, free weights, exercise bands, digging, lifting, carrying shopping, circuit training, and step aerobics. I took up weight training a few months ago and can highly recommend it. Paradoxically, I find it rather relaxing. If you do take up weight training I'd recommend getting some professional instruction on how to lift safely.

Examples of ways to improve balance include: sideways walking, heel-to-toe walking, one-leg stand, back leg raises, and side leg raises. Practicing standing from sitting, yoga, and tai chi will also improve balance. Always consider safety, but you can incorporate some of these into your daily routine. Why not stand on your left leg when you brush your teeth in the morning and on your right leg when you brush them at night? Or include some sideways walking or back leg-raises as you vacuum to music around the house.

Strength and balance exercises are particularly important as we get older as they will keep muscles and bones strong and will help to reduce the risk of falling. Improving strength and balance can also help to reduce the fear of falling, which is a common reason why people become less physically active and limit their own activity so that they miss out on opportunities for social contact in later life.

9. Rest and recovery

Any fitness regime needs to include time for rest and recovery. Sleep, hydration, and nutrition are all important aspects of recovery. Don't get too obsessive about exercising all of the time and don't forget to stretch. Warm up before you exercise; include dynamic stretching before your activity sessions and static stretching afterward. Be careful how you schedule your day. Be realistic about what you can achieve. Don't place unrealistic demands on yourself. Make sure you incorporate rest days.

10. Play

Have fun. Play upbeat music in the house while you prepare dinner or do the chores. Or simply put on your favorite song and dance around your kitchen, bedroom, or office. It's hard to resist the temptation to dance or move in time to the music.

Play an active sport. Taking up a team sport gives you the added bonus of spending time in the company of others. Play actively with your kids, grandkids, nieces, or nephews. It will be good for them, too. Find a tennis or golf partner and play together. Getting physically active with friends can increase the enjoyment. You're more likely to stick at it if you have fun.

I started this chapter with the reminder that as children we run and jump for the sheer joy of it. I want to end with a reminder to have fun. Too often we see exercise as something that we have to do. Another chore, an unpleasant "grin and bear it" sort of activity. I'd like to suggest simply grinning while you exercise. This small attitude adjustment can have real benefits. Smiling while you exercise may help you to relax, reduce muscle tension, improve the efficiency of your performance, and make your workout feel less effortful and more enjoyable. You can read more about the brain-health benefits of smiling and a positive attitude in the next chapter.

PHYSICAL—PART TWO

Goals—Action Plan—Personal Profile

Set your goals, devise your action plan, and create your personal profile for Physical.

Brain Health Goals: Physical

Answering the following questions, using your Physical Log and IPAQ scores, will help you to set physical goals to boost your brain health.

Q1. Physical activity

Based on the *Assessment: Physical Log* and *Assessment: IPAQ* my physical activity category is:

High ☐   Moderate ☐   Low ☐

> **Physical Goal No. 1**
>
> I want to increase my activity category ☐
>
> No action required: my physical activity levels are optimum for my health ☐

Q2. Physical activity pattern

Looking at my *Assessment: Physical Log* and *Assessment: IPAQ* scores I have:

A good balance between moderate activity and vigorous activity:
   Yes ☐   No ☐

Based on my usual activities I have:

A good balance between aerobic, strength, and balance activity:
   Yes ☐   No ☐

Physical Goal No. 2

I want to increase my levels of
moderate activity ☐   vigorous activity ☐   walking ☐

I want to increase my
strength ☐   balance ☐   aerobic activity ☐

No action required: I'm happy with my physical activity pattern ☐

Q3. Sitting

Seated-based work should be broken up with standing work and vice versa. To begin with, the most recent recommendations are to break up sitting spells throughout the working day, so as to accumulate at least two hours every day of standing and light activity (light walking) during working hours with the ultimate aim to progress to four hours every day.

Based on your *Assessment: Physical* and *Assessment: IPAQ* scores
My weekday sitting total is ____

My average sitting total is (weekday sitting total divided by five (assuming you work a five-day week)

Physical Goal No. 3

I want to break up long spells of sitting ☐

I want to reduce the overall time I spend sitting each day ☐

No action required: I sit for a healthy amount of time and don't sit for long periods without breaks ☐

Completing the table on the next page using the information from your Physical Goals will help you to characterize your current healthy habits and prioritize any physical habits that need fixing. Tick the box that applies then enter any items that need fixing into the Brain Health Action Plan on page 203.

	Healthy	Needs fixing	Priority*
Moderate levels of activity			
Vigorous levels of activity			
Walking			
Sitting			
Work-related			
Transport-related			
Home-related			
Leisure-related			
Aerobic			
Muscle-strengthening			
Bone-strengthening			
Balance			
Other			

* High, medium, or low

Brain Health Action Plan: Physical

Enter your physical habits that need fixing items from the table on the previous page into the Brain Health Action column in the table overleaf. Indicate whether the action is attainable with relative ease in the short term (quick fix) or will require more time and effort to achieve (long term). The ten tips that you have just read should help you to break each action into practical steps. Prioritize the actions in the order you would like to work on them (1 = tackle first).

Brain Health Action	Order	Steps	Quick fix	Long term

Personal Profile: Physical

Using your scores in the **Brain Health Goals: Physical** section as a guide, complete this table. Indicate whether your scores are healthy, borderline, or unhealthy. From that you can determine whether your current pattern of behavior is a brain-healthy asset or a risk that could compromise your brain health and make you vulnerable to dementia in later life. Finally, indicate the aspects that you would like to fix, improve, or maintain and prioritize them for inclusion in your Brain Health Plan in Chapter 9.

Aspect	Healthy	Borderline	Unhealthy	Asset	Risk	Maintain	Improve	Fix	Priority
Activity level									
Activity type									
Sitting									
Total									

100 Days to a Younger Brain

PROGRAM DAYS 22–30: GETTING PHYSICAL

You should now have a clear understanding of your current physical activity levels, your personal goals, and the actions that you need to take to benefit your brain health. You will combine your physical activity profile with the other profiles that you will create as you complete this program to produce your overall Brain Health Profile in Chapter 9. You will also select at least one of your physical actions to add to your overall Brain Health Plan.

100-DAY DIARY

You can record the steps that you are taking toward your program goals in the 100-Day Diary at the back of the book. For example:

- I got off the bus two stops early today.
- I danced around the kitchen when my favorite song came on the radio.
- I took the stairs instead of the lift at work today.
- I set an alarm on my phone to remind me to stand and walk about every hour instead of sitting at my desk all day.

You can also celebrate your healthy habits by recording them in your 100-Day Diary.

8

Adjust Your Attitude

"There is nothing either good or bad,
but thinking makes it so."
William Shakespeare—*Hamlet*

ATTITUDE—PART ONE

Your brain has the ability to change itself physically and functionally in response to your experiences and to your behavior. This natural neuro-plasticity means that your brain can also morph in response to your thinking. You can shape your brain not only by the actions you choose to take but also by the way that you think about and approach life.

When it comes to brain health, changing your behavior is not enough. You also need to manage your thoughts, attitudes, and perceptions and do so with care. Your attitude to aging, to memory, and even to happiness can actually change your brain and shape your future to the benefit or detriment of your brain health.

If you face each day with the attitude that you are who you are and cannot change you may be depriving yourself of opportunities to boost your brain health.

Changing how you feel about aging may actually change how you age. The practical tips in this chapter will help you to make life-changing attitude adjustments and the assessments will give you personal insights that will help you transform your attitude to benefit your brain health. You will use this information to create your personal attitude profile, set goals, and devise an attitude action plan in Part Two of this chapter.

This chapter explains how smiling, ditching aging stereotypes, and adopting a positive attitude to aging can not only improve your memory but also lengthen your life.

Quick Question: Attitude

When was the last time that you smiled? __/__/___ Time _____

How often do you smile every day? _____

Brain Gains: How Does Attitude Impact Brain Health?

Smile

Memory processing can be enhanced by reward. When we see a smiling face it feels rewarding to us. If you want people to remember you, smile. We remember smiling faces better than surprised, angry, or fearful faces. We can quickly recall the names of people who smile. This enhanced memory for smiling faces occurs because of the effect that your brain's reward regions have on memory regions.

The reward system in the brain evolved to motivate us to engage in behaviors such as eating food, drinking water, and having sex—activities that keep us alive and promote the survival of our species. To enhance survival, the reward system in the human brain drives desire, craving, and motivation, triggering positive emotions like pleasure to maximize our interactions with things that benefit us.

When you eat something, let's say a "triple-decker sandwich," special neurons in a specific area of your brain involved in reward, release the neurotransmitter dopamine, giving you a surge of pleasure. To ensure that you will repeat this "eating" behavior the reward centers in your brain are connected to the areas in your brain that control memory and behavior. Remembering that eating that triple-decker sandwich made you feel good will make you more likely to eat it again.

In addition to maximizing our contact with things that benefit our survival the brain also needs to minimize our interaction with things that can cause us harm. The fear system in the human brain evolved to keep us safe. There is overlap between the reward and fear networks in your brain. At the most fundamental level, through the activation of these systems you feel fear and you learn associations so that your behaviors are incentivised, conditioned, reinforced, rewarded, and/or punished. This means that you are likely either to approach or avoid food, things, objects, events, people, activities, and situations depending on whether they have given you pleasure or pain. One thing that sets us apart from other animals is our ability to pursue rewards that may be months or even years away, like saving for our own home, studying for exams, working toward promotion, or completing a 100-day brain health program.

Pleasure centers

The core structures of your reward system are located in your "limbic brain," which evolved to manage fight or flight. You have read a lot about its main structures—the hippocampus, hypothalamus, and amygdala—in this book because of their involvement in learning, memory, emotions, mood, fear, and stress. This limbic system is also involved in the release of hormones and in managing unconscious bodily functions like appetite and emotional states.

The neurotransmitter dopamine plays a critical role in the control of the reward and pleasure centers in your brain, responding to everything from food, to sex, to addictive drugs. Dopamine also plays a role in memory and movement, allowing you to recognize and move toward or "approach" rewards so that you can pick up that sandwich, open your mouth wide enough to get around all three delicious layers, then chew and swallow it down. When you encounter something rewarding, your brain responds by increasing the release of dopamine. While dopamine is found all over your brain there is a coherent dopamine reward and motivation system that involves a number of key areas in your brain, including your prefrontal cortex.

Your orbitofrontal cortex is part of your prefrontal cortex and, as the name suggests, it sits at the front of your brain just above your eye sockets (orbits). It is well connected with the parts of your brain that process information from your senses (e.g., the visual cortex) and with structures in your brain involved in emotion (e.g., the amygdala) and in memory (e.g., the hippocampus). Your orbitofrontal cortex helps to determine how rewarding something is. In essence, it codes the things that you taste, smell, touch, hear, and see in terms of their reward value so you find that triple-decker sandwich more rewarding than a spinach salad, for example.

Approachable faces

In the context of memory for faces and names, your orbitofrontal cortex and your hippocampus become significantly activated when you successfully encode a face with the correct name. Interestingly these successful memory activations are greater for happy faces than they are for faces with no discernable expression.

We use facial expressions to help us to make decisions about whether to avoid or approach a person in a social situation. If a person's face is angry we may feel anxious and walk away to avoid them. If we encounter a happy smiley face we will be more inclined to approach the person. Smiling faces tend to activate the hippocampus and the left frontal region of the brain. In contrast, frowning or threatening faces tend to activate right frontal and dorsal midbrain regions. These patterns of brain activation are associated with what we call "approach–avoidance" motivation.

So why is this relevant to brain health? Well, approach-related brain activation is associated with optimal brain functioning and with optimal levels of neuroplasticity and neurogenesis. Avoidance-related brain activation suppresses the growth of new neurons most probably to limit the impact of stressful or negative events on the brain. Our ability to think and process information also tends to be enhanced by reward. As a general rule we tend to thrive in social situations where social interactions are based on the communication of positive emotions.

Social interactions facilitate the growth of new neurons through increased neural activity. To survive in society we have evolved in a way that allows us to communicate our intentions, motivations and emotions through posture, movements, and facial expressions. Your face is a powerful communication tool with a repertoire of facial expressions that can influence the behavior of others. People are likely to view your smiling face as attractive, kind, trustworthy, and even familiar.

Assessment: Happiness

For each of the following statements and/or questions, please circle the point on the scale that you feel is most appropriate in describing you.

1. In general, I consider myself:

Not a very happy person					A very happy person	
1	2	3	4	5	6	7

2. Compared with most of my peers, I consider myself:

Less happy					More happy	
1	2	3	4	5	6	7

3. Some people are generally very happy. They enjoy life regardless of what is going on, getting the most out of everything. To what extent does this characterization describe you?

Not at all					A great deal	
1	2	3	4	5	6	7

4. Some people are generally *not* very happy. Although they are not depressed, they never seem as happy as they might be. To what extent does this characterization describe you?

Not at all					A great deal	
1	2	3	4	5	6	7

Reprinted by permission from Springer Nature: Social Indicators Research, 46 (2) p. 137, "A measure of subjective happiness: preliminary reliability and construct validation" Lyubomirsky, S., & Lepper, H. Copyright © 1999, Kluwer Academic Publishers and from Professor Sonja Lyubomirsky, University of California Riverside.

What your score means

Item	How to score	Your score
1	Your score is the number you circled	
2	Your score is the number you circled	
3	Your score is the number you circled	
4	Score as follows 7 = 1, 6 = 2, 5 = 3, 4 = 4, 3 = 5, 2 = 6 and 1 = 7	
Total	Add your scores for the 4 items	
Your score	Divide your total score by 4	

Average scores differ depending on a number of factors, but generally speaking an average on the happiness scale runs from 4.4 to 5.5—if your score is greater than 5.6 you are happier than average, if you score less than 4.4 you are less happy than average.

Transfer your score to Question 2, Part Two of this chapter (Brain Health Goals: Attitude).

Social rewards

Even though our reward centers are activated by money, the people most satisfied with life tend not to be those with the most money but rather those with the strongest social connections. The brain experiences physical pleasure when we are socially rewarded. This can happen when someone rewards us with a smile, when we cooperate with other people, when we receive recognition from others or when our reputation is given a bit of a boost. The power of social reward becomes evident when you realize that when given a choice most people are more motivated by social rewards than monetary rewards.

Natural anti-depressant

When you flash your pearly whites the feel-good factor kicks off in your brain and dopamine, serotonin, and endorphins are released. Smiling activates reward circuits in your brain. Thanks to its starring role in pleasure and reward, the release of dopamine increases your feelings of happiness. The serotonin released by your smile acts as a natural antidepressant and the endorphins serve as a natural pain reliever. Smiling makes you feel happy and relaxed; it boosts your brain health by releasing hormones that lower your blood pressure, boost your immune function and protect you against stress, depression, and anxiety.

Happiness trigger

Smiling isn't just the consequence of a good mood, it can be the cause of one, too. We tend to think of smiling as something spontaneous, an involuntary action that is triggered by happiness or joy, but the scientific fact of the matter is that smiling can trigger happiness, too. By simply turning the corners of your mouth up rather than down you can boost your brain health. Despite its incredible complexity, or maybe because of it, your brain allows itself to be fooled by a manufactured smile into releasing the chemicals that make you feel happy.

You will recall from Chapter 5 that mirror neurons fire both when we observe another person carry out an action and when we take part in that action ourselves. When you see someone smile your mirror neurons will stimulate your own smiling. Humans are natural mimics. We have an inherent and involuntary tendency to automatically imitate other people's facial expressions. The interesting thing is that this mimicry isn't just superficial. By that I mean that it involves more than just the areas of your brain that activate muscle movements. Facial mimicry activates brain regions that trigger emotional states. When you see a smiling face it won't just make you respond with a superficial smile, it will evoke real feelings of happiness within you.

Right or left hemisphere

Optimism and pessimism are ways of thinking about the future that run along a continuum of positive or negative outcomes. Our tendency toward optimism or pessimism is context specific. For example, we may feel that every romantic relationship we enter is ultimately doomed but we always expect to succeed at work. Our tendency can also change from time to time. We all have rose-tinted, blue-sky days where we feel highly optimistic about everything and everyone, and what I call low-ceiling days where clouds descend and we can see nothing but doom and gloom. The assessment overleaf measures generalized optimism versus pessimism.

Assessment: Life Orientation Test

Respond honestly to the ten statements below. Try not to let your response to one statement influence your responses to the others. There are no correct or incorrect answers. Answer according to your own feelings, rather than how you think "most people" would answer.

A = I agree a lot

B = I agree a little

C = I neither agree nor disagree

D = I disagree a little

E = I disagree a lot

		A, B, C, D, or E
1	In uncertain times, I usually expect the best.	
2	It's easy for me to relax.	
3	If something can go wrong for me, it will.	
4	I'm always optimistic about my future.	
5	I enjoy my friends a lot.	
6	It's important for me to keep busy.	
7	I hardly ever expect things to go my way.	
8	I don't get upset too easily.	
9	I rarely count on good things happening to me.	
10	Overall, I expect more good things to happen to me than bad.	

What your score means

		Score
1	A = 4, B = 3, C = 2, D = 1, E = 0	
2	A = 0, B = 0, C = 0, D = 0, E = 0	
3	A = 0, B = 1, C= 2, D = 3, E = 4	
4	A = 4, B = 3, C = 2, D = 1, E = 0	
5	A = 0, B = 0, C = 0, D = 0, E = 0	
6	A = 0, B = 0, C = 0, D = 0, E = 0	
7	A = 0, B = 1, C= 2, D = 3, E = 4	
8	A = 0, B = 0, C = 0, D = 0, E = 0	
9	A = 0, B = 1, C= 2, D = 3, E = 4	
10	A = 4, B = 3, C = 2, D = 1, E = 0	
	My total score	

The Life Orientation Test (LOT-R) measures generalized optimism versus pessimism. There is no cut-off score for optimism or pessimism but as a general rule the average score is 14–15. If you score higher than this you are more optimistic than average, and if you score lower than this you are more pessimistic than average.

Transfer your score to Question 1, Part Two of this chapter (Brain Health Goals: Attitude).

Optimism is associated with better health and a longer life. People tend to respond to the optimist's expectation of being liked by liking them. Your attitude influences how resilient you will be, especially when bad things happen. Optimists tend to be tougher, more persistent, and indeed more resilient in the face of adversity.

Optimists tend to bounce back from bad experiences because they believe that bad things are temporary; they see a single setback rather than a final defeat. Optimists also tend not to generalize from the specific to the universal. By that I mean that they tend to see a "one-off" barrier where a pessimist will see something that will undermine everything they try to do going forward.

Optimists are also more likely to acknowledge multiple causes and less likely to blame themselves than pessimists. This means that pessimists often quit, stop trying, and lose hope, which can lead to depression. In contrast, optimists create more opportunities for themselves. They make a brighter future because they tell themselves the future will be brighter.

Of course, every experience that you have involves both hemispheres of your brain. Having said that, your right hemisphere is more attuned to negative information in your environment while your left hemisphere is more attuned and more receptive to positive information. Eye-tracking studies show that optimists gaze at negative or unpleasant images less than pessimists. The optimist's attention is biased toward the positive in their environment.

Who is in control?

If you believe that the events in your life are controlled by outside forces you have what's referred to as an external locus of control. In contrast, if you believe that you are the master of your own destiny you have what's referred to as an internal locus of control. What you believe about your ability to control important aspects of your life will shape your attitude.

People with an external locus of control tend to see events as passively happening to them, determined by luck, fate, or chance. In contrast, people with an internal locus of control feel in control of their own destiny and see themselves as playing a very active role in their successes and failures and in shaping their life events. They believe in their own ability to shape their future and influence the world and the people around them.

An internal locus of control tends to be associated with activation of the left hemisphere while an external locus of control tends to be associated with right hemisphere activation. Pessimists have a tendency toward an external locus of control while optimists tend toward an internal locus of control. Anxiety is closely linked to our perception of control, so people with an external locus of control tend to be prone to anxiety. In contrast, people with an internal locus of control tend to be happier, less stressed, and less depressed, which is a boon for your brain health. The questionnaires that follow assess depression and will give you an indication of whether you tend toward an internal or external locus of control.

Assessment: Locus of Control

For each question tick the statement (a or b) that best describes how you feel.

- ☐ 1a. Many of the unhappy things in people's lives are partly due to bad luck.
- ☐ 1b. People's misfortunes result from the mistakes they make.
- ☐ 2a. One of the major reasons why we have wars is because people don't take enough interest in politics.
- ☐ 2b. There will always be wars, no matter how hard people try to prevent them.
- ☐ 3a. In the long run, people get the respect they deserve in this world.
- ☐ 3b. Unfortunately, an individual's worth often passes unrecognized no matter how hard he tries.
- ☐ 4a. The idea that teachers are unfair to students is nonsense.
- ☐ 4b. Most students don't realize the extent to which their grades are influenced by accidental happenings.

☐ 5a. Without the right breaks, one cannot be an effective leader.

☐ 5b. Capable people who fail to become leaders have not taken advantage of their opportunities.

☐ 6a. No matter how hard you try, some people just don't like you.

☐ 6b. People who can't get others to like them don't understand how to get along with others.

☐ 7a. I have often found that what is going to happen will happen.

☐ 7b. Trusting to fate has never turned out as well for me as making a decision to take a definite course of action.

☐ 8a. In the case of the well-prepared student, there is rarely, if ever, such a thing as an unfair test.

☐ 8b. Many times exam questions tend to be so unrelated to course work that studying is really useless.

☐ 9a. Becoming a success is a matter of hard work; luck has little or nothing to do with it.

☐ 9b. Getting a good job depends mainly on being in the right place at the right time.

☐ 10a. The average citizen can have an influence in government decisions.

☐ 10b. This world is run by the few people in power, and there is not much the little guy can do about it.

☐ 11a. When I make plans, I am almost certain that I can make them work.

☐ 11b. It is not always wise to plan too far ahead because many things turn out to be a matter of luck anyway.

☐ 12a. In my case, getting what I want has little or nothing to do with luck.

☐ 12b. Many times we might just as well decide what to do by flipping a coin.

☐ 13a. What happens to me is my own doing.

☐ 13b. Sometimes I feel that I don't have enough control over the direction my life is taking.

Score 1 point for each of the following: 1a, 2b, 3b, 4b, 5a, 6a, 7a, 8b, 9b, 10b, 11b, 12b, 13b—for all others score 0

Locus of Control Score ___

What your score means

Scores range from 0–13.

A high score indicates that you have an external locus of control.

A low score indicates that you have an internal locus of control, which is better for brain health.

Transfer your score to Question 5, Part Two of this chapter (Brain Health Goals: Attitude).

Assessment: Depression

Once you have answered all of the questions, turn to the next page to get the values for each of your choices. Enter them in the score column

Tick the box that best describes how you have felt over the last week. During the past week…	Rarely or none of the time < 1 day	Some or a little of the time 1–2 days	Occasionally or a moderate amount of time 3–4 days	All of the time 5–7 days	Score
1. I was bothered by things that don't usually bother me.					
2. I did not feel like eating, my appetite was poor.					
3. I felt that I could not shake off the blues, even with help from my family.					
4. I felt that I was just as good as other people.					
5. I had trouble keeping my mind on what I was doing.					
6. I felt depressed.					
7. I felt that everything I did was an effort.					
8. I felt hopeful about the future.					
9. I thought my life had been a failure.					
10. I felt fearful.					
11. My sleep was restless.					
12. I was happy.					
13. I talked less than usual.					
14. I felt lonely.					
15. People were unfriendly.					

Tick the box that best describes how you have felt over the last week. During the past week...	Rarely or none of the time < 1 day	Some or a little of the time 1–2 days	Occasionally or a moderate amount of time 3–4 days	All of the time 5–7 days	Score
16. I enjoyed life.					
17. I had crying spells.					
18. I felt sad.					
19. I felt that people disliked me.					
20. I could not "get going."					
Total					

What your score means

Item	Rarely or none of the time < 1 day	Some or a little of the time 1–2 days	Occasionally or a moderate amount of time 3–4 days	All of the time 5–7 days
4, 8, 12, and 16	3	2	1	0
All other items	0	1	2	3

Add all items together to get your total score ___

While a score of 16 or higher is considered depressed* it is important to reiterate that this is not a diagnostic tool. If you are concerned that you might be depressed, regardless of your score, it is important that you seek help sooner rather than later.

Transfer your score to Question 4, Part Two of this chapter (Brain Health Goals: Attitude).

Aging attitudes

We all know what aging is, don't we? Or do we? Well, we are certainly familiar with the outward signs of aging, such as graying hair and wrinkling skin. Even if we haven't experienced these manifestations yet ourselves, thanks to advertising we can't help but know about them or at least know what product to buy to prevent or hide these "terrible" abominations that await our older selves!

---

* Depression (Centre for Epidemiological Studies—Depression (CES-D Scale))

Chronological age

It's a bit of an understatement to say that in Western society we have become obsessed with counting up the years since birth. Is aging really just about that, just about our chronological age? Certain life exposures and life choices mean that your biological age might actually be greater or less than your chronological age. This means that the age of your body, including your brain, might be greater or less than your numerical age as a consequence of numerous factors, such as whether you smoke, exercise, or eat a healthy diet.

Is aging just illness?

Maybe the status of our health is more relevant to aging than our chronological age? Over a lifetime it's usual to have survived a number of infections and as we get older we are at increased risk of medical conditions and chronic diseases. Is aging just illness, the accrued effects of illness, or the increased risk of illness? If that is the case mustn't that mean that we have at least some control over the aging process when we make choices that influence our health and our exposure to risk of illness and disease?

Roles

Maybe when we talk about aging we are really talking about our changing role in society. As we progress through life our roles change and society expects us to behave and be treated in ways appropriate to these roles. We move from being someone's infant, to being a student, then an employee, maybe we will be someone's boss, someone's mum or dad, aunt, uncle, grandparent, and so on. For many roles in society there are age expectations. For example, we expect an athlete to generally be under the age of thirty, while we expect a high court judge to be double that age.

Restrictions

Society often imposes arbitrary age restrictions that prevent individuals from engaging in certain activities or enforce them to cease specific activities. Depending on the country or culture you might not be legally entitled to marry, vote, have sex, or drink alcohol until you have reached the age of sixteen, seventeen, eighteen, or twenty-one. Retirement is a concept hugely associated with age, where many people perfectly capable of continuing to contribute to the workforce are prevented from doing so once they hit sixty-five, based on nothing other than an arbitrary decision about retirement age made by Otto von Bismarck in 1883.

Expectations and experience

Our responsibilities and sense of worth can also change with societal roles, and this influences the way we think. Is aging really about conforming to societal expectations? Do we act older than we really are? Do we conform to societal expectations by slowing down and taking it easy when in reality we are not only capable of doing more but after a few months of retirement would really relish the opportunity to contribute to society and feel useful?

So what do we really mean by aging?

Well, probably all of the above. Aging doesn't just suddenly start at sixty-five, it's been going on your entire life. How you age is dependent on a multitude of factors—some beyond your control and others very much within your control. We all age in different ways.

The aging process is influenced by so many factors, including our medical history, our genetic heritage, the society we live in, our life experiences and exposures, how we perceive ourselves, and even our attitude to aging. As a consequence of this interplay between dynamic factors the aging process doesn't follow the same trajectory for everyone. This means that factors like your mother's diet, the quality of the air that you breathe, the length of your telomeres (protective tips on your DNA), and even whether you have a positive or negative view of aging will influence the path that aging takes.

Living longer

In trying to understand why some people live longer in good health than others, scientists often turn their attention to SNPs (pronounced snips—*single-nucleotide polymorphisms*), which are like typographical errors, or typos, in your genetic code.

These little mistakes in DNA sequences can generate biological differences in people by causing alterations in the recipes for proteins in their genes. In turn those differences can impact on things like how long a person will live, their physical appearance, their health, and their susceptibility to disease.

The SNPs associated with longevity in people who have reached the age of 100 are negatively linked to Alzheimer's disease and heart disease. This means that aging without developing a disease may well be linked to the absence of risk factors for heart disease and for Alzheimer's disease, rather than being linked to the longevity genes.

Your lifestyle, the things you choose to eat, and the toxins that you are exposed to, including drugs of abuse and stimulants like nicotine, will impact on how long you live, how many of those years you will spend in good health, and may also influence the development of neurodegenerative diseases like dementia.

Thanks to scientific advancement we are now living longer. Sweeping changes in people's behaviors have improved health and reduced the incidence of early death. But we don't just want to live longer, we want those extra years to be spent in good health, preferably in possession of our full mental faculties. Reaching the age of eighty without chronic disease is a relatively rare occurrence but one that is linked to SNPs that are involved in cognitive performance, which opens up the possibility that brain health and cognition may actually be determinants of healthy aging.

The power of perceptions

The number of years since your birth is, of course, a factor in aging, but the point I'm making is that it's not the only factor. Each of us is unique and the way that our brain ages will reflect our personal history, heritage, culture, experiences, life choices, and our attitudes.

I find this knowledge very empowering because it means that we do have some control over how we age.

For sure, you can't control your genetic heritage or change your life history but you can shape your future by changing how you think today. Something simple like adjusting your attitude to aging itself can pay big dividends. For example, having a positive view of aging will buy you an extra few years of life. *Older adults with positive self-perceptions of aging live, on average, seven and a half years longer than older*

adults with less positive ones! That's a pretty big payoff for a shift in attitude. Taking the next assessment will tell you whether you have a positive or negative attitude to aging.

Assessment: Attitude to Aging

Enter the score for the statement that best reflects how you feel where:

SD = Strongly disagree, D = Disagree, N = Neither agree nor disagree, A = Agree, SA = Strongly agree

	Statement	SD (1)	D (2)	N (3)	A (4)	SA (5)
1	It is a privilege to grow old.					
2	There are many pleasant things about growing older.					
3	Old age is a depressing time of life.					
4	I don't feel old.					
5	I see old age mainly as a time of loss.					
6	I have more energy now than I expected for my age.					
7	As I get older I find it more difficult to make new friends.					
8	It is very important to pass on the benefits of my experiences to younger people.					
9	I want to give a good example to younger people.					
10	I feel excluded from things because of my age.					
11	My health is better than I expected for my age.					
12	I keep as fit and active as possible by exercising.					

What your score means

The most important thing is not to total up all scores. There is no total score, as there are three separate parts to this questionnaire: Psychological Loss (PL), Psychological Growth (PG), and Physical Change (PC).

To figure out your own score for:

PL: add items 3 + 5 + 7 + 10. PL Score ___

PG: add items 1 + 2 + 8 + 9. PG Score ___

PC: add items 4 + 6 + 11 + 12. PC Score ___

Each maximum total score is 20, as the individual questionnaire items score 1–5.

A higher score for PL in particular indicates a negative attitude.

For very rough guidance, people in good health report scores for PL, PG, and PC on average as 9, 14, and 14.

If you want to figure out a "positive" attitude to aging profile, it would be higher scores on Psychological Growth and Physical Change and lower scores on Psychological Loss. Evidence from a number of different studies from across the world suggest that Psychological Loss scores, and to an extent Physical Change scores, are negatively affected by depression levels or when people are physically unwell or if they rate their health as poor.

Transfer your score to Question 3, Part Two of this chapter (Brain Health Goals: Attitude).

Our stereotyped view of aging can change our behavior, which in turn can impact on our brain health. Our preconceptions can exert an influence that makes us behave as we believe older people should behave and may lead to us ceasing activities, like engaging in stimulating occupations or taking physical exercise or taking on new challenges, that could help to protect us from illness, disease, and decline in our cognitive and physical functioning.

The internalizing of aging stereotypes begins in childhood. As early as four years of age, children are able to pick out the oldest person from pictures of people of varying ages. They also associate the oldest adults with being helpless, passive, and incapable of caring for themselves. This means that in the first few years of life we learn and unconsciously assimilate stereotypes about aging. These stereotypes are reinforced in adulthood and become self-stereotypes as we age, then ultimately we behave according to our internalized stereotype. Which is not good when you consider that many grown-ups see aging as synonymous with failing mental function.

So perhaps when we talk about aging we are really talking about psychological aging; how we perceive ourselves and how others perceive us.

Our attitudes to aging are so powerful that simply switching older adults' perceptions of aging to more positive perceptions improves physical function to the same level as a six-month exercise program!

Older, wiser, happier

We are surrounded by so much negativity about aging that I think it is really important to acknowledge that growing older isn't all unrelenting despondency. For starters, happiness increases with age. Older people are happier than middle-aged people and younger people. Now it is true that levels of happiness do decrease in very late life but they never return to the levels of unhappiness that we experienced in early adulthood. This could be because we are actually happier or because we become better at synthesizing happiness as we get older.

Life may have taught us the benefits of putting a positive spin on things. It is also possible that being faced with the reality that we have lived longer than we have yet to live helps us to focus on what matters most to us, making us less likely to waste precious time on trivial things that add little value to our lives. With age our perception of time changes. Our appreciation of its preciousness may lead us to make choices that enrich our emotional experiences in ways that make us feel happier.

Our levels of worry, stress, and anger also decrease with age. Plenty of other things get better with age, too. Older people are much better at resolving conflicts, possibly because life experience brings with it knowledge, wisdom, and expertise, so they more easily understand different sides of an argument and are better at predicting what might happen next and more willing to seek compromise.

Light-bulb moment

Your brain is comprised of a series of interacting networks. While you chat with a friend a couple of those networks are actively engaged. The network in your frontal lobes will allow you to pay attention to what your friend is saying, process the information and then formulate a response. When your mind wanders or when you are not actively focused on a task, a particular group of brain regions, called the default mode network, actually become more active.

Your ability to reflect on feelings such as whether you are happy or not is associated with this default mode network. If I wanted to measure your default mode network I'd fit you with an EEG cap and tell you to close your eyes and not think of anything in particular while I recorded the electrical activity in your brain.

It might surprise you to learn that your brain becomes even more active when you are in that daydreaming state than it does when you are actively paying attention. We think that insight, problem-solving, and creativity stem from the interaction between this resting state network and the executive network in the brain.

I'm sure you've had a light-bulb moment where you have a great idea, or a Eureka moment where you suddenly figure out a problem. Your idea or solution has emerged because this network probes your long-term memory to find associations among the Aladdin's cave of riches that is your life experiences and exposures. This mesh of information might help you to solve the problem at hand or give you insight into your level of happiness or give rise to creativity and new ideas.

When you have to make big decisions I'm sure someone has advised you to sleep on it. Neuroscience supports the "sleep on it" adage. Semantic memory refers to the general knowledge of the world that you have accumulated and abstracted from your life experiences. This knowledge in your brain underlies your ability to use language, engage socially, and mentally project yourself back and forward in time.

Over the course of your life you have built up a wealth of information in your brain, so throw the information that is relevant to the problem at hand into the mix, leave it to marinate and your brain will find the magic ingredients in your semantic networks. More often than not your brain will present you with the solution the next morning after a good night's sleep.

Wisdom is one of the greatest gifts of age and experience.

No-Brainer: Smile, it's free, it's simple, and it boosts brain health.

Brain Drains: What Happens When You Have a Negative Attitude to Aging?

Negative attitudes to aging abound in Western society. It's not surprising since we are bombarded with negative messages about aging. Aside from advertisements everywhere that equate being older with being unattractive, older adults are portrayed as forgetful, dependent, helpless, and unproductive. The reality of the matter is that the majority of older people are self-sufficient with a wealth of experience, time, and talent to offer society.

When it comes to the entertainment industry, older people, if they appear at all, are frequently little more than caricatures. Often portrayed as dependent, lonely, disagreeable individuals with multiple physical and mental ailments, this kind of stereotyping leads to ageism and a failure to acknowledge diversity. All old people are not the same; in fact, populations of older people are more complex and more diverse than those of younger people, mainly because they have lived longer and have had more opportunity for diverse life experiences.

Negative stereotypes and negative perceptions of older people impact us as we age in very real ways. As we become older we have poorer employment prospects, are more likely to be excluded in social situations and, rather shockingly, are less likely to receive the same medical treatment as younger adults even when that treatment would be effective.

Unfortunately, negative stereotypes don't just bounce off us. We absorb them and internalize them and when we apply them to ourselves we may end up restricting our own roles and expectations at work and in our lives in a way that can accelerate the aging process and negatively impact on our health, including our brain health. Negative self-perceptions can also impact on our psychological well-being, mood, confidence, and our physical ability.

When it comes to aging, our perceptions are pretty powerful. Over-fifties who have negative perceptions of aging lose mental sharpness. In a research situation immediate declines in cognitive function are recorded when older adults are primed to have negative self-perceptions of aging. To explain, priming can just involve the use of negative aging stereotype words (such as senile, dependent, incompetent).

Rather alarmingly, one study showed that when cognitively normal older adults are primed to have negative self-perceptions in relation to their age it results in a decline in their cognitive functioning to a level below the cut-off on tests designed to detect dementia. A cut-off score is a bit like a pass or fail mark in an exam; above the cut-off is considered in the normal range, below the cut-off is considered an indication of dementia.

How you think about yourself in terms of your age even influences your memory performance. This means that people who classify themselves as older and who expect memory to decline with age actually perform more poorly on memory tests. People with negative perceptions of aging not only lose mental sharpness but also tend to gradually withdraw from social activities, which, given the importance of social connection, is not good for brain health.

Some older adults become physically frail in later life. They lose weight and muscle strength, they become slower on their feet, tend toward inactivity and feelings of exhaustion. Frailty is associated with risk for multiple health problems and a higher risk of developing dementia. Frail people with negative perceptions of aging have poorer mental function when compared to people who are not frail. But the good news is that frail people with positive perceptions of aging have the same level of mental ability as their non-frail counterparts.

Note the good news

Bad stereotypes about aging or indeed about anything are quicker to form and more difficult to eradicate than good ones. We seem to be more attuned to the negative in our lives than the positive. As children we are more affected by the red "x" beside the misspelled words in our spelling test than we are by the tick next to the correct ones. We rarely forget criticism, losing money, or falling out with friends. Bad health impacts on our happiness more than good health. Generally speaking, negative events and experiences tend to have a greater impact on us than positive ones.

It seems that we have an innate predisposition to pay attention or give more weight to the negative. From an evolutionary perspective this makes sense for survival; being attuned to bad things makes it more likely that we will survive threat and danger. We need to pay urgent attention and act more quickly to potentially bad outcomes to ensure survival.

While ignoring a possible positive outcome may leave us with a sense of missed opportunity, ignoring a potentially negative outcome could leave us injured, ill or no longer alive. Our brain also seems to cognitively process bad things more thoroughly than good things. It also needs to make sure that we retain information about "bad" events so as to minimize their likely reoccurrence.

Our evolutionary history means that the human brain automatically prioritizes bad news. Your brain doesn't have a mechanism for noting the good news, so you need to make a conscious effort to count your blessings. Interestingly, the most mentally sharp older adults show a tendency to direct their attention and memory toward positive information rather than negative. Cultivating a slight bias toward optimism without losing sight of reality can bring about a bounty of bonuses, including a reduced chance of clinical depression, a stronger immune system, greater adaptability in the face of challenge, and a longer life.

> **No-Brainer**: Keep negative perceptions about your age and your mental abilities in check.

Summary

- When we see a smiling face it feels rewarding to us.
- The neurotransmitter dopamine pays a critical role in the control of the reward and pleasure centers in your brain.
- Social interactions facilitate the growth of new neurons through increased neural activity.
- When you flash your pearly whites the feel-good factor kicks in within your brain. Dopamine, serotonin, and endorphins are released. Smiling activates reward circuits in your brain increasing your feelings of happiness.
- The serotonin released by your smile acts as a natural anti-depressant and the endorphins serve as a natural pain reliever.

- Smiling makes you feel happy and relaxed. Smiling boosts your brain health by releasing hormones that lower your blood pressure, boost your immune function, and protect you against stress, depression, and anxiety.
- Smiling isn't just the consequence of a good mood, it can be the cause of one, too.
- Certain life exposures and choices mean that your biological age might actually be greater or less than your chronological age.
- How you age is influenced by multiple factors, some of which are under your control.
- Older adults with positive self-perceptions of aging live, on average, seven and a half years longer than older adults with less positive ones!
- Older people are happier than both middle-aged and younger people.
- Our levels of worry, stress, and anger also decrease with age.
- Relax and let your default mode network solve problems and present you with great ideas.
- Wisdom is one of the greatest gifts of age and experience.
- Applying negative stereotypes to ourselves may lead to us restricting our own roles and expectations in a way that can accelerate the aging process.
- Over-fifties who have negative perceptions of aging lose mental sharpness.
- How you think about yourself in terms of your age influences memory performance.
- The most mentally sharp older adults show a tendency to direct their attention and memory toward positive information rather than negative.

Brain Changers: What You Can Do

Your attitude has a very real impact on how you age. Smiling more, cultivating optimism, and adjusting your attitude won't just boost your brain health, it will bring a whole host of benefits.

TEN PRACTICAL TIPS TO ADJUST YOUR ATTITUDE

1. Adjust your attitude to aging.
2. Add gratitude to your attitude.
3. Increase your odds.
4. Cultivate optimism.
5. Take control.
6. Be inspired by amazing agers.
7. Banish senior moments.
8. Marinate.
9. Act on ageism.
10. Smile.

1. Adjust your attitude to aging

Check your language; avoid phrases like "back in my day" or "when I was in my prime." Frame these expressions more positively. Rather than referring to yourself as a lesser person now than when you were younger, consider simpler statements like "When I was in my twenties..."

Be proud of getting older. Put a positive spin on it, remember that older means wiser and happier. Acknowledge the reality that most older adults live well and independently. Despite the impression the media gives, only 5 percent of adults over sixty-five live in nursing homes or other forms of assisted living.

Check your own prejudices and question whether you are making assumptions about your own or others' abilities based on age.

2. Add gratitude to your attitude

Start a gratitude journal. Get in the habit of writing down one thing every day that you can be grateful for. This will help you to counteract your brain's natural tendency to pay attention to the negative and will help you to focus on the positive things in your life. Even when life seems pretty grim the discipline of writing just one positive thing each day will help you realize that although terrible things befall us sometimes, there is always something that we can be grateful for.

When life threw me one curveball more than I thought I could cope with, forcing myself to find one thing to write each day helped me to find perspective. Things weren't going my way but that was no reason to wallow in my own misery. I had hands and feet and food and I could hear and see and...

You get the point. It sounds a bit preachy but it is practical, doable, and it does work. Give it a go. A gratitude journal is a simple way to train a positive outlook. It forces you to focus on the positive aspects of your life, which can increase serotonin levels in your brain. The serotonin influences dopamine, which makes you feel good and when you feel good chances are you'll feel happy, too.

Alternatively, send a thank-you email or make a point of expressing your gratitude to at least one person every day. Saying thank-you is more than just good manners, it actually makes you happier. Feeling grateful activates areas in your brain that release dopamine. Saying thank-you to the bus driver, the office cleaner, or that random person who holds the door open for you increases activity in your dopamine circuits, leading to a greater sense of enjoyment from your social interactions.

Giving is good, too. Give your time and give others a helping hand. You can recharge yourself by thinking of and helping others.

3. Increase your odds

How well you and your brain age is influenced by a multitude of factors. The choices that you make influence how the cells in your body and your brain perform, repair, and survive. Increase your odds of aging well by managing your health, staying connected to your community, and by continually engaging in ongoing personal development. What you get out of life and how well you age depends a great deal on what you put into life.

Switch your perspective of aging from a passive process that simply happens to you to an active one over which you can exert considerable control. Don't let age stop you from investing in your future. Take exercise, make healthy choices, and continue to contribute to society. Nurture your talents and keep on learning and developing new skills and abilities. Keep learning, keep growing, and keep setting goals. It is vital to keep your skin, even if it is wrinkled, in the game.

4. Cultivate optimism

Some people have optimism-pessimism "set points" where they consistently lean toward one extreme or the other. While a healthy dose of optimism tempered with some plain old realism has genuine health benefits, it is important to acknowledge that our brain has evolved to support both optimism and pessimism. While it is beneficial to cultivate optimism it shouldn't be confused with a need to completely erase pessimism.

There is a fine balance between both optimism and pessimism that holds the key to successfully navigating the world in a way that allows you to welcome challenges without being reckless or learn from adversity rather than being defeated and immobilized by it. A cost-benefit analysis may help you to decide whether optimism is the way to go in any given situation. When the stakes are high, optimism might not be the best policy. A bit of pessimism in risky circumstances might help to save your life, your marriage, or your career.

If you lack a natural tendency toward optimism, don't worry—it can be learned. It just requires some conscious mindful effort and the involvement of the left hemisphere of your brain.

Your point of view can be trained. Become conscious of when you appraise something as negative and try to reappraise it by focusing on the positive aspects. When you do this it will activate regions in the left hemisphere of your brain. Become aware of the voice in your head. What stories are you using to "explain" the events unfolding in your life? Ask yourself if you are being pessimistic. Are you seeing permanence in something that will pass? Are you catastrophising? Are you blaming yourself to the exclusion of all other causes? Check your thoughts and try to consciously reframe them in a more positive light.

5. Take control

You can shift your attitude and sense of control by watching your language and recognizing that you can exercise choice. When you hear yourself say "I have no choice," question it. Have you explored the options? Do you really have no other option? It can help to ask others for ideas. Sometimes we can control more than we realize. Choose what is best for you, even if it is Hobson's choice. If your choices are limited, even reframing your viewpoint from "I have no choice" to "I don't like my choices but I will do x, y, z because it is in my best interest" will help you to accept or change your situation.

While lots of things in life are actually beyond our control, adjusting our attitude to them can help us to cope with them, freeing us up to focus on the things that we can control. A realistic view of what you can and can't control coupled with an internal locus of control can make you feel empowered and emboldened to set goals and take on challenges, both of which enhance the quality of your life and the health of your brain.

6. Be inspired by amazing agers

Optimism, resilience, and perseverance characterize "super-agers," with many demonstrating a never-say-die attitude and a need to have a sense of control. Ageist stereotypes and the general invisibility of older people in the media, and indeed in society, means that we have to look a little harder to find inspirational healthy brain agers, but they are there.

I experienced pure joy when I first met our university's oldest student, ninety-eight-year-old Joe Veselsky. He was interesting, inspirational, and entertaining. He refused to use the lift even though that meant that both he and I had to climb several flights of stairs. I simply loved that he had to leave the event I was hosting early to catch his lecture. I am fortunate that my work in the community places me in the company of older adults frequently, so that I am constantly inspired.

In the public sphere late-life achievers and healthy-brain agers can be found in numerous disciplines. To whet your appetite, Italian neurologist Rita Levi-Montalcini who won the Nobel Prize in Physiology or Medicine, continued to work in her lab until after she turned 100, helping to further our understanding about dementia. Frenchwoman Jeanne Calment, who died at age 122, maintained a sharp brain for decades after "normal" life expectancy. Even though her hearing and sight deteriorated, she entertained reporters and visitors with witty retorts. One of my favorite broadcasters, Sir David Attenborough, recently fronted a TV wildlife series at the age of ninety-two. Fashion icon Iris Apfel recently became the oldest person ever to have a Barbie doll made after her!

Michelangelo changed the world of art with his paintings and sculptures, and some of his greatest works came after he'd turned seventy. At eighty-eight, Michelangelo drew up the architectural plans for the magnificent church of Santa Maria degli Angeli e dei Martiri. Frank Lloyd Wright completed New York's Guggenheim Museum at age eighty-nine and continued teaching until his death in 1959. American folk artist "Grandma Moses" embarked on a twenty-five-year painting career at the age of seventy-six. At eighty-five, Coco Chanel was the head of a fashion design firm, and at ninety-one Adolph Zukor was chairman of Paramount Pictures. Verdi was in his seventies when he composed *Otello* and *Falstaff*. Churchill, Goethe, Shaw, Maugham, and Tolstoy all produced literary works in their eighties. Edna O'Brien is still writing novels at eighty-seven and Diana Athill has embarked on another literary adventure at the age of 100.

In Britain, retired dental surgeon Charles Eugster, author of *Age is Just a Number*, took up bodybuilding at the age of eighty-seven. Then at ninety-five he took up sprinting and went on to become world champion in his age category. Ernistine Shepherd (eighty-two) began working out at 56 and holds the Guinness World Record as oldest female bodybuilder. In New York City, Tao Porchon-Lynch (ninety-nine), was declared the world's oldest yoga instructor when she was ninety-three. She has had a long and varied career as a couture model, an actress, a film producer, television executive, and a publisher. A competitive ballroom dancer, she appeared on *America's Got Talent* in 2015. Her motto is "there is nothing you cannot do."

7. Banish senior moments

In the late 1990s the ageist but socially acceptable attribution *senior moment* entered our vocabulary to describe the phenomenon of a brief lapse in memory or other cognitive function. When people over sixty-five are reminded of the link between age and cognitive decline they perform poorly on memory tests. Even individuals in late middle age underperform on memory tests when they are implicitly reminded of the relationship between age and memory decline. These research findings underline the impact that our preconceptions, even when they are wrong, can have on our actual functioning.

So don't make self-deprecating jokes about "senior moments" and keep in mind that decline in cognitive function is not inevitable. If you unconsciously or subconsciously accept that decline is inevitable, or even if you joke about "senior moments," you might get yourself caught up in a negative feedback loop and end up fulfilling your own prophesy.

8. Marinate

If a problem doesn't have to be solved today or a decision isn't needed immediately, don't force it. Let the information marinate in your brain for a bit. Allow the non-conscious parts of your amazing brain to find the solution for you. Let your default mode network do its job. How many times have you woken up with the solution to a problem that you'd wrestled with the previous day to no avail? How many times have you woken up and realized that the quick decision you'd made the previous day might not have been the wisest?

Sometimes it can take longer than one sleep, so trust that your default mode network is working away in the background, leave it to marinate and let it do its job, probing your semantic networks, the different parts of the brain that have encoded the experiences that you've lived through. Apply the same principles to creative pursuits and the flavor of your ideas and insights will be enhanced by time spent marinating among the networks of your brain soup.

Sometimes there is just too much going on in your brain. Your brain gets overcrowded so it's important to kick back and relax a little to give your default mode network some space to work.

9. Act on ageism

Big changes happen when lots of people do little things. Ageism is so deeply embedded in our society that I personally believe that the only way that we can eradicate it is if each and every one of us takes responsibility to stamp it out one step at a time. My suggestions are:

- Next time you attend a social gathering, make a point of engaging with someone at least twenty years older or twenty years younger than you. Check yourself for prejudices as you chat, and dismiss these thoughts in favor of openness and a willingness to discover more about the person than their age.

- Challenge negative stereotypes. Write a letter or email to the paper, TV show, or advertiser next time you encounter ageism. While some of us do become frail and dependent with age it's a much smaller proportion than the media would have us believe. As a society it's time we asked the media to start painting a more accurate picture of older adults that acknowledges reality.
- Try to see the person and not the age. Remember, ageism occurs in both directions, so be careful of stereotyping young people.
- Call out any age discrimination you come across. Be brave. You don't have to be confrontational. You can very gently and politely point out why something is ageist.

10. Smile

Finally, my favorite brain-health tip of all is to smile. It's free and it boosts brain health. It gives birth to new brain cells and encourages changes in areas of the brain associated with learning and memory. It makes your brain more flexible, more resilient, and better able to cope when challenged by stress.

Smiling releases hormones that make you feel good, it lowers blood pressure, boosts immune function, and protects against stress, depression, and anxiety. The simple act of smiling sends messages to your brain that can make you happy even if you are not.

Smile at least five times a day, even or especially if you don't feel like it. Start and end your day with a smile. Spread the happiness and the health benefits by sharing at least one smile every day with someone else. It's contagious and can lead to laughter, which is nature's stress-buster.

Feel free to do whatever you wish with the other two smiles.

ATTITUDE—PART TWO

Goals—Action Plan—Personal Profile

Set your goals, devise your action plan, and create your personal profile for Attitude.

Brain Health Goals: Attitude

Answering the following questions will help you to set attitude-adjustment goals to boost your brain health. *You will find a completed sample in the back of the book.*

Q1. Optimism–Pessimism

Based on *Assessment: Life Orientation Test* score, I am:

- ☐ More optimistic than average
- ☐ Less optimistic than average
- ☐ About average

Attitude Goal No. 1

I want to cultivate a more optimistic approach to life ☐

I want to temper my optimism with a little more realism ☐

No action required: I have a healthy level of optimism ☐

Q2. Happiness

My *Assessment: Happiness* score is _____; this suggests that I am:

- ☐ More happy than average
- ☐ Less happy than average
- ☐ About average

Attitude Goal No. 2

I want to feel happier ☐

I'd like to smile more ☐

I'd like to laugh more ☐

No action required: I am happy ☐

Q3. Attitude to Aging

Base your answer on your *Assessment: Attitude to Aging*.

I have a positive attitude to aging: Yes ☐   No ☐

Attitude Goal No. 3

I want to challenge my own perceptions of aging:
Yes ☐   No ☐

I want to develop a more positive attitude to aging:
Yes ☐   No ☐

No action required: I have a healthy attitude to aging ☐

Q4. Depression

My *Assessment: Depression* score is ___

My score indicates that I may be depressed: Yes ☐   No ☐
My score is a good indication of how I feel ☐
My score is not a good indication of how I feel ☐

Attitude Goal No. 4

I want to take action to address my mood: Yes ☐   No ☐

No action required: my mood is positive and
well balanced ☐

Q5. Locus of control

Based on *Assessment: Locus of Control* I have an:

☐   Internal locus of control
☐   External locus of control

Attitude Goal No. 5

I want to shift my sense of control toward an
internal locus ☐

No action required: I have an internal locus of control ☐

Completing the table below using the information from your Attitude Goals will help you to characterize your current healthy habits and prioritize any stress habits that need fixing. Tick the box that applies then enter any items that need fixing into the Brain Health Action Plan on the next page.

	Healthy	Needs fixing	Priority*
Attitude to aging			
Focus on positives in my life			
Gratitude for the positives in my life			
Setting goals			
Actively controlling how I age			
Cultivating optimism			
Sense of control			
Actively making choices			
Choice of language			
Act on ageism			
Smiling			
Other			

* High, medium, or low.

Brain Health Action Plan: Attitude

Enter your attitude habits that "need fixing" items from the table on the previous page into the Brain Health Action column in the table below. Indicate whether the action is attainable with relative ease in the short term (quick fix) or will require more time and effort to achieve (long term). The ten tips that you have just read should help you to break each action into practical steps. Prioritize the actions in the order you would like to work on them (1 = tackle first).

Brain Health Action	Order	Steps	Quick fix	Long term

Personal Profile: Attitude

Using your scores in the **Brain Health Goals: Attitude** section as a guide, complete this table. Indicate whether your scores are healthy, borderline, or unhealthy. From that you can determine whether your current pattern of behavior is a brain-healthy asset or a risk that could compromise your brain health and make you vulnerable to dementia in later life. Finally, indicate the aspects that you would like to fix, improve, or maintain, then prioritize them for inclusion in your Brain Health Plan in Chapter 9.

Aspect	Healthy	Borderline	Unhealthy	Asset	Risk	Maintain	Improve	Fix	Priority
Optimism									
Happiness, smiling, and laughter									
Attitude to aging									
Mood									
Locus of control									
Total									

100 Days to a Younger Brain

PROGRAM DAYS 31 AND 32: ADJUSTING YOUR ATTITUDE

You should now have a clear understanding of your attitudes, your personal goals, and the adjustments that you need to make to benefit your brain health. You will combine your attitude profile with the other profiles that you have produced as you worked through this program to achieve your overall Brain Health Profile in Chapter 9. You will also select at least one of your attitude actions to add to your overall Brain Health Plan.

100-DAY DIARY

You can record the steps that you are taking toward your program goals in the 100-Day Diary at the back of the book. For example:

- I monitored my thoughts and tried to switch some negatives to positives.
- I bought the top I liked rather than the one I felt was most suited to my age.
- I started a gratitude journal.
- I smiled five times today.

You can also celebrate your healthy habits by recording them in your 100-Day Diary.

9

Build Your Bespoke Brain

"It is not the strongest of the species that survive, nor the most intelligent, but the one most responsive to change."
Charles Darwin

Congratulations for making it this far, you are now ready to devise your bespoke brain-health investment strategy. You now know that key lifestyle changes and activities that reduce risk or offer protection can easily be incorporated into your daily routine.

You need to develop a daily brain-health habit because you now understand that investing time in your brain health today will add life to your brain, and protect it against future decline and the effects of disease. The small things you do each day can make a difference.

You will increase your chances of success if you link the actions in your plan to things that are fundamentally important to you and intrinsic to your life. Ask yourself why you want to improve your brain health. Is it because you want to live independently in your own home? Maybe it's because you want to continue making a meaningful contribution to your community or want to play an active role in the lives of your children and grandchildren. Or perhaps you want to remain in possession of your full faculties and be able to share your wit and wisdom with those who matter to you most. Whatever your reason, keep it in mind as you devise and implement your plan.

By reading this book you have taken a very important first step by increasing your knowledge of neuroscience, dementia risk, and opportunities for investment in brain health. Through self-assessment you have accumulated important information about yourself, your current habits, your assets and risks. It's now time to use this personal information to create an honest Brain Health Profile that will inform your initial Brain Health Plan and your longer-term brain-health investment strategy to minimize dementia risk and maximize the return on your investment.

Because your brain is unique, crafted by the experiences that you offer it and the demands that you place on it, a "one-size-fits-all" plan won't wash for brain health. You need to create a brain-health investment mix that is based on your personal goals, your current brain health situation, the timeline that you are working within (e.g., your age, your life stage), and the amount of risk factors that you have and can modify.

As you develop your plan remember the importance of diversity. In addition to building a mix of investments across sleep, stress management, social engagement, mental activity, heart health, physical activity, and attitude you also need to incorporate variety within these investments (such as physical activity—aerobic exercise, muscle strengthening, balance, and sitting less).

Remember, brain health is a long-term investment. The Brain Health Plan that this book helps you to develop is the first and a hugely important step in a long-term strategy that aims to improve your brain health one day at a time. Regularly revisiting and updating your profile and Brain Health Plan will allow you to track progress, take account of changing circumstances, and let you see whether you need to rebalance your "asset" mix or reconsider some of your individual investments.

You have nothing to lose and everything to gain. Confidence is key to success. Devise your strategy then implement it one day at a time. When it comes to brain health, it is entirely within your power to transform your debts into assets by making conscious brain-healthy choices and incorporating simple changes to your daily life.

PROGRAM DAYS 33 AND 34:
BUILD YOUR BRAIN HEALTH PROFILE
AND BESPOKE BRAIN HEALTH PLAN

Brain Health Profile

Complete the Brain Health Profile table on the next page to create an overview of your brain-health assets and risks and get a clear snapshot of the current state of your brain health—this is your Brain Health Profile. *You will find a completed sample in the back of the book.*

Brain Health Plan

Next complete your Brain Health Plan. The overarching aim of your Brain Health Plan should be to increase your assets and reduce your risks across each of the six brain-health factors (Sleep, Stress, Social/Mental, Heart, Physical, and Attitude).

Select one priority goal for each lifestyle factor from the individual action plans that you created in Chapters 3, 4, 5, 6, 7, and 8.

If you think it is feasible and realistic you can include more than one goal per lifestyle factor. If you decide to do this, my advice would be to select a long-term goal and a quick win rather than two long-term goals. If you have a particularly healthy category (for instance, you manage stress well) you can choose to devote extra effort to a lifestyle factor that needs more work (such as physical activity).

This is your personal journey. Your brain is unique and so your Brain Health Plan needs to be unique to you.

You will find a completed sample in the back of the book.

Brain Health Profile

Transfer the total scores from your Personal Profiles in Chapters 3 to 8 into the corresponding rows opposite and total each column. Your overarching aim should be to increase your assets and reduce your risks for each of the lifestyle factors. *You will find a completed sample in the back of the book.*

Category	Healthy	Borderline	Unhealthy	Asset	Risk	Maintain	Improve	Fix	Priority
Sleep									
Stress									
Social/ Mental									
Heart									
Physical									
Attitude									
Total									

Brain Health Plan

Category	Goal	Action	Steps	Target date
Sleep				
Stress				
Social/ Mental				
Heart				
Physical				
Attitude				

Put Your Plan into Action

PROGRAM DAYS 35–100: GET THE BRAIN-HEALTH HABIT

I have allowed sixty-six days to embed the brain-health habit into your daily life. Of course, sixty-six days is the average time it takes to build a habit so that means that some of the brain-healthy behaviors that you want to introduce will need less than sixty-six days and some will need more than this time to become habits.

How long it takes to form a new habit will depend on multiple factors, some of which will be very personal to you and to the behaviors that you want to eradicate and replace. Some actions will be easier to implement than others.

Consider the long game—brain health is for life. Don't attempt to change everything at once but rather prioritize the things that you would like to improve and work on them during your first 100 days until they become automatic.

To break old habits you have to work hard at first to override your existing pattern of behavior, but with time repeating the new behavior will strengthen the connections in your brain so that your newly trained behavior becomes your new habit. Tacking the new behavior onto an existing routine may help you to stick to your plan.

Focusing on something strengthens it. Try to focus on developing the new behavior rather than resisting the old one. Rehearse the new habit in your head. Simply imagining the new behavior can help to build a new habit.

When a new brain-healthy habit has become routine you can revisit your action plans and select a new goal to add to your overall ongoing Brain Health Plan.

Track your achievements

Use the table overleaf to record your achievements. The journey to brain health is more of a marathon than a sprint so to keep motivated it is important to record your achievements along the way. Record each step and action that you complete toward your goal.

If you prefer, you can keep track in an Excel file or record your achievements in a traditional pen and paper notebook or journal.

You might consider sharing your journey in a brain-health blog or on social media using *#BrainHealth*.

Taking stock in this way will help you to embed brain health into your daily routine. Sharing your intention and progress publicly can be a good way to motivate you, keep you on track, and encourage you to be inventive and innovative in the things that you do along your 100-day journey to brain health.

Brain Health Achievement Record

Achievement	Date achieved	Benefits/comments

And finally, remember...

- Look after your brain as routinely as you look after your teeth.
- You need your brain for everything, so brain health matters.
- Everyone with a brain needs to consider brain health.
- Your brain is constantly changing.
- Your behaviors, your experiences, and the lifestyle choices that you make can shape it at any age.
- It's never too early or too late to invest in brain health.
- Your brain is plastic and can change throughout your life.
- Your brain is resilient and has the capacity to build reserves.
- What you do, and what you don't do, influences how well your brain functions now and how resilient it can be when faced with challenges such as aging, injury, or disease.
- Key lifestyle changes, activities, and attitudes that protect your brain function, slow brain aging, and reduce dementia risk can easily be incorporated into your daily life.

Activity	Attitude	Lifestyle
Get physical	Manage stress	Cherish sleep
Stay social	Think positive	Love your heart
Go mental	Smile	Protect your head

100-Day Diary

The key aim of keeping this 100-Day Diary is to help you to make brain health an integral part of your daily life. The brain-healthy actions or choices that you record in the diary don't have to be fancy or life-changing. In fact, they don't even have to be new.

In the first instance while you are building your profile over the first thirty days, I would suggest that you focus on recording and celebrating the things that you already do each day that are good for brain health.

Making a daily entry will serve the dual purpose of getting you to think about your brain health every day while also familiarizing yourself with your own brain-health assets. It's a bit like taking stock or building an asset map that will help you to highlight which lifestyle factors are most in need of your attention.

As you progress through the book you might take on board some of the tips in each chapter and begin to record these together with some of the "quick fix" actions that you identify in Chapters 3 to 8.

Once you have built your bespoke Brain Health Plan your aim should be to increase your assets across your entire Brain Health Profile by completing activities every day that tick all of the categories (Sleep, Stress, Social, Mental, Heart, Physical, and Attitude).

You will find that many activities will address more than one factor. For example, attending your book club will address both social and mental factors. Walking to the club will allow you to check the physical activity box, too, and so on—you get the picture. I've entered some milestones into the 100-Day Diary.

As you read through this book you will discover that you are already doing lots of things that are good for your brain health, so start your journey by celebrating that. During your first week focus on your current assets and record your existing brain-healthy habits.

Record at least one thing each day but don't be afraid to record several	
Day	Brain-healthy choice/action
1	
2	
3	
4	
5	
6	
7	Milestone: sleep profile & plan completed

	Tick all of the factors that your brain-healthy action addresses						
	Sleep	Stress	Social	Mental	Heart	Physical	Attitude

Have you identified any sleep-improvement "quick-wins" that you could implement this week to improve the quality of your sleep?

Record at least one thing each day but don't be afraid to record several	
Day	Brain-healthy choice/action
8	
9	
10	
11	
12	
13	
14	Milestone: stress profile & plan completed

Have you identified any stress-improvement "quick-wins" that you could implement this week to better manage stress or to find your personal stress sweet spot?

Record at least one thing each day but don't be afraid to record several	
Day	Brain-healthy choice/action
15	
16	Milestone: mental & social profile & plan completed
17	
18	
19	
20	
21	

	Tick all of the factors that your brain-healthy action addresses						
	Sleep	Stress	Social	Mental	Heart	Physical	Attitude

	Tick all of the factors that your brain-healthy action addresses						
	Sleep	Stress	Social	Mental	Heart	Physical	Attitude

Have you identified any social- or mental-activity improvement "quick wins" that you could implement this week?

Record at least one thing each day but don't be afraid to record several	
Day	Brain-healthy choice/action
22	
23	Milestone: heart health profile & plan completed
24	
25	
26	
27	
28	

How are you doing on physical activity? Were you surprised to learn that the recommended 150 minutes per week must be in addition to your baseline levels of physical activity?

Record at least one thing each day but don't be afraid to record several	
Day	Brain-healthy choice/action
29	
30	Milestone: physical activity profile & plan completed
31	
32	Milestone: attitude profile & plan completed
33	Milestone: brain health profile completed
34	Milestone: bespoke brain health plan completed
35	

Now that you have a clear picture of your current Brain Health Profile it's time to ramp things up a little. Your diary entries should reflect the steps in your bespoke Brain Health Plan. Let your action plan inform your choices and actions each day.

Tick all of the factors that your brain-healthy action addresses							
	Sleep	Stress	Social	Mental	Heart	Physical	Attitude

Tick all of the factors that your brain-healthy action addresses							
	Sleep	Stress	Social	Mental	Heart	Physical	Attitude

Record at least one thing each day but don't be afraid to record several	
Day	Brain-healthy choice/action
36	
37	
38	
39	
40	
41	
42	

You don't have to record everything but it is important to make at least one entry every day as this will help to reinforce the brain-health habit. Focus on the new habits you are trying to embed and aim to check as many lifestyle-factor boxes as you can each day.

Record at least one thing each day but don't be afraid to record several	
Day	Brain-healthy choice/action
43	
44	
45	
46	
47	
48	
49	

	Tick all of the factors that your brain-healthy action addresses						
	Sleep	Stress	Social	Mental	Heart	Physical	Attitude

	Tick all of the factors that your brain-healthy action addresses						
	Sleep	Stress	Social	Mental	Heart	Physical	Attitude

Congratulations, it's the halfway point, a good time to take stock again. How are you doing? Are you making progress? Did you take on too much? Perhaps you underestimated your abilities and haven't challenged yourself enough. Revisit your Brain Health Plan and make adjustments accordingly. Don't forget to note the date on which you attain any of your goals in your Brain Health Plan. Keep recording your achievements.

Record at least one thing each day but don't be afraid to record several	
Day	Brain-healthy choice/action
50	
51	
52	
53	
54	
55	
56	

	Tick all of the factors that your brain-healthy action addresses						
	Sleep	Stress	Social	Mental	Heart	Physical	Attitude

This week take some time to focus on sleep. Record any progress that you have made. Have a look back at the **Sleep Log** that you completed in week one, has your sleep improved? Are you still on target to achieve your goal? If not, see whether you need to adjust your behavior or your goal. If you have already achieved your sleep goal and feel ready for another challenge, consider adding a new sleep goal to your overall plan.

Record at least one thing each day but don't be afraid to record several	
Day	Brain-healthy choice/action
57	
58	
59	
60	
61	
62	
63	

	Tick all of the factors that your brain-healthy action addresses						
	Sleep	Stress	Social	Mental	Heart	Physical	Attitude

This week take time to focus on stress. Record any progress that you have made. Have a look back at the **Stress Log** you completed in week two, have things changed? Are you still on target to achieve your goal? If not, see whether you need to adjust your behavior or your goal. If you have already achieved your stress goal and feel ready for another challenge, consider adding a new stress management goal to your overall plan.

Record at least one thing each day but don't be afraid to record several	
Day	Brain-healthy choice/action
64	
65	
66	
67	
68	
69	
70	

Tick all of the factors that your brain-healthy action addresses						
Sleep	Stress	Social	Mental	Heart	Physical	Attitude

This week take some time to focus on social and mental activity. Record any progress that you have made. Have a look back at the social and mental profile completed in Chapter 5, have things changed? Are you still on target to achieve your goal? If not, see whether you need to adjust your behavior or your goal. If you have already achieved your goal and feel ready for another challenge, consider adding a new goal to your overall plan.

Record at least one thing each day but don't be afraid to record several	
Day	Brain-healthy choice/action
71	
72	
73	
74	
75	
76	
77	

	Tick all of the factors that your brain-healthy action addresses						
	Sleep	Stress	Social	Mental	Heart	Physical	Attitude

This week take some time to focus on your heart. If you don't know your stats, make an appointment to get your BP, cholesterol, and sugar levels tested. Record any progress that you have made. Have a look back at the **Food Log** you completed in week one, have things changed? Are you still on target to achieve your goal? If not, see whether you need to adjust your behavior or your goal. If you have already achieved your goal and feel ready for another challenge, consider adding a new heart-health goal to your overall plan.

Record at least one thing each day but don't be afraid to record several	
Day	Brain-healthy choice/action
78	
79	
80	
81	
82	
83	
84	

Tick all of the factors that your brain-healthy action addresses						
Sleep	Stress	Social	Mental	Heart	Physical	Attitude

This week take some time to focus on your physical activity. Record any progress that you have made. Are you achieving the recommended exercise levels? Are you still on target to achieve your goal? If not, see whether you need to adjust your behavior or your goal. If you have already achieved your goal and feel ready for another challenge, consider adding a new physical goal to your overall plan.

Record at least one thing each day but don't be afraid to record several	
Day	Brain-healthy choice/action
85	
86	
87	
88	
89	
90	
91	

Tick all of the factors that your brain healthy action addresses							
Sleep	Stress	Social	Mental	Heart	Physical	Attitude	

This week take some time to focus on your attitude. Record any progress that you have made. Are you smiling and laughing more? Have you noticed a change in your attitude to aging? Are you still on target to achieve your goal? If not, see whether you need to adjust your attitude or your goal. If you have already achieved your goal and feel ready for another challenge, consider adding a new attitude goal to your overall plan.

Record at least one thing each day but don't be afraid to record several	
Day	Brain-healthy choice/action
92	
93	
94	
95	
96	
97	
98	

	Tick all of the factors that your brain-healthy action addresses						
	Sleep	Stress	Social	Mental	Heart	Physical	Attitude

Almost there. On your hundredth day take some time to reflect on your journey, complete the assessments on page 274, and celebrate your successes by recording them here.

Record at least one thing each day but don't be afraid to record several	
Day	Brain-healthy choice/action
99	
100	

Congratulations!

	Tick all of the factors that your brain-healthy action addresses						
	Sleep	Stress	Social	Mental	Heart	Physical	Attitude

Post-Program Assessments

A. Repeat the Verbal Fluency Assessment from Chapter 3.

Set a timer for one minute and record yourself as you name as many animals you can as quickly as possible.

Listen back and record your total correct score.

B. Assessment: Memory, Health, and Well-Being

You will need a pen and paper to complete this task.

1. Read the following list, concentrating on each word for a few seconds.

1a. Remember these words:

Car	Paper	Cabbage	Table
Window	Bread	Summer	Hat
Grass	Van	Phone	Nail

1b. Now close the book and write down as many words as you can recall.

   Your score is the total number of words that you recalled correctly

   ___

2. How would you rate your general health at the present time?

   Excellent ☐　　Very good ☐　　Good ☐　　Fair ☐　　Poor ☐

3. How would you rate your overall sense of well-being at the present time?

   Excellent ☐　　Very good ☐　　Good ☐　　Fair ☐　　Poor ☐

4. How would you rate your day-to-day memory at the present time?

   Excellent ☐　　Very good ☐　　Good ☐　　Fair ☐　　Poor ☐

How do your scores today compare to your scores in Chapter 3 when you completed the assessments before you began the program?

Now that you have completed the program you can re-take some of the assessments in Chapters 3–8, this will allow you to update each lifestyle profile to see and celebrate the progress that you have made on each brain health factor over the last 100 days.

You can use this information to create your new Brain Health Profile on the next page.

Day 101: Update Your Brain Health Profile

Category	Healthy	Borderline	Unhealthy	Asset	Risk	Maintain	Improve	Fix	Priority
Sleep									
Stress									
Mental/ social									
Heart									
Physical									
Attitude									
Total									

Samples

Sample: Chapter 3
Brain Health Action Plan: Sleep

Action	Order	Steps	Quick fix	Long term
Remove technology from my bedroom and limit use of light-emitting devices close to bedtime	1	Find a new place to charge my laptop and phone	x	
		Don't bring devices into the bedroom ever		x
		Don't work from bed		x
		Buy an old-school alarm clock	x	
Get a more regular bedtime	3	Based on my schedule, establish bedtime	x	
		Set a bedtime alarm on my phone	x	
		Try it for a week even if I don't actually sleep		x
Try to get at least 7.5 hours of sleep a night	5	Keep tabs on the hours I'm sleeping		
		See if any of the changes are making a difference		x
Develop a wind-down routine	2	Read suggestions for wind-down	x	
		Try a few different things		x
		Try having a bath at night		
		Stop using Netflix to relax late at night	x	
		Try to go back to reading print books at night	x	x
Develop a regular sleep schedule	4	Try to be disciplined about going to bed and getting up on the same time, even at weekends		x
Avoid eating after 7:30 p.m.	6	Schedule mealtimes into my day	x	
		Prepare some meals on the weekend so I can just heat them up after work	x	

Sample: Chapter 3
Personal Profile: Sleep

Aspect	Healthy	Borderline	Unhealthy	Asset	Risk	Maintain	Improve	Fix	Priority
Duration	x			x			x		
Schedule		x			x			x	x
Quality	x			x	x				
Disturbance	x			x	x				
Barriers			x		x			x	x
Total	3	1	1	3	2	2	1	2	2

Note: Two priority actions entered in Brain Health Plan.

Sample: Chapter 4
Assessment: Stress Log

Day	Time	Duration	Stressor	Location	Activity	Level	Regular	Coping strategy
Mon	17:55	10 mins	Waiting for parking at gym	Gym	Getting in line to park at gym	1	Yes	none
Tues	09:55	30 mins	Lost property dept.	Phone	Speaking with lost property agent at airport	2	no	Breathed deeply and told myself that getting angry with the agent might make my situation worse
Weds								
Thurs								
Fri								

Sample: Chapter 4
Brain Health Action Plan: Stress

Brain Health Action	Order	Steps	Quick fix	Long term
Spend less time working	1	Do an audit on what I spend my time working on	X	
		Minimize time-consuming unimportant work		X
		Start saying no or giving more realistic deadlines		X
		Do not respond/read emails after working hours	X	
		Respond to emails only at 2 time points daily	X	
		Schedule meetings more realistically		X
Spend more time smiling and laughing	2	Make a conscious effort to smile every day	X	
		Identify things/people that make me laugh	X	
		Make an effort to spend more time with people I have fun with		X
		Try to see the funny side more often		X
Spend more time outside	3	Factor "outside" breaks into my day	X	
Pursue my interest in photography	4	Spend time outside photographing birds, nature, flowers on weekends		X

Sample: Chapter 5
Brain Health Action Plan: Social and Mental

Brain Health Action	Order	Steps	Quick fix	Long term
Engage in more challenging leisure activities	1	Watch less TV	x	
		Keep an eye out for local exhibitions/talks	x	
		Try to do something "cultural" at least once a month		x
		Instead of meeting friends/family for lunch/coffee or drinks suggest going to exhibition/public talk/theater	x	
Increase my social network	2	Make more of an effort to meet people more regularly than I have been doing		x
		Accept invitations to events more often		x

Sample: Chapter 6
Heart: Food Log

(Use common objects to help estimate portions. For example a 75 g/3 oz steak = deck of cards, and a cup of rice = tennis ball)

	Day1	Day 2	Day 3	Day 4	Day 5	Day 6	Day 7
Day	Thurs						
Breakfast	Oatmeal Almond milk						
Lunch	Can of tuna, lettuce, tomato, onion, cucumber						
Dinner	Sea bass, peas, broccoli, butter, cup of rice						
Snacks	Banana						
Water	6 glasses						
Fluids	1 green tea						
Alcohol	Gin & tonic						
Comments	I think I did well today. Although I could feel my resolve weaken even after just one gin.						
Fat	low						
Salt	low						
Sugar	In fruit & tonic						
Cigarettes	19						

Sample: Chapter 6
Brain Health Action Plan: Heart

Brain-Health Action	Order	Steps	Quick fix	Long term
Lower my blood pressure	2	Talk to my doctor about management and treatment options	x	
		Quit smoking		x
		Lose weight		x
		Exercise regularly		x
		Reduce the amount of salt in my diet	x	
Quit smoking	1	Make a list of all the reasons why I want to quit	x	
		Pick a date I want to quit by	x	
		Open a savings account for the money I'll save		x
		Look up supports online to help me quit	x	
		Take up a hobby that will keep my hands busy		x

Sample: Chapter 7
Physical Log

Type	Life Domain	Mon Mins	Tues Mins	Weds Mins	Thurs Mins	Fri Mins	Sat Mins	Sun Mins	Days	Total Mins	MET minutes
Vigorous	Work	0	0	0	0	0	0	0	0	0	Vigorous total mins (work + leisure) x 8
	Leisure	40	0	45	0	30	0	30	4	145	Vigorous MET minutes = 1,160 (145 x 8)
Moderate	Work	0	0	0	0	0	0	0	0	0	Moderate total mins (work + home + leisure) x 4
	Home	15	0	30	20	25	20	0	5	110	
	Leisure	0	30	0	0	0	0	0	1	30	Moderate MET minutes = 560 (140 x 4)
Walking	Work	0	0	0	0	60	60	30	3	150	Walking total mins (work + transport + leisure) x 3.3
	Transport	0	0	0	0	0	0	0	0	0	
	Leisure	0	0	0	0	0	30	0	1	30	Walking MET minutes = 594 (180 x 3.3)
Total MET minutes											**Vigorous + Moderate + Walking** 1,160 + 560 + 594 = 2,315
Sitting											**Weekdays sitting total**
	Work	480	540	0	0	200	200	240	7	1660	
	Other	240	300	200	240	200	240	200	7	1662	

Sample: Chapter 7
Assessment: IPAQ, Category Calculation

High-intensity level criteria

- Vigorous-intensity activity on at least three days, achieving a minimum total physical activity of at least 1,500 MET minutes/week.

Sample score—vigorous activity MET = 1,160, Days = 4: doesn't qualify
OR

- Seven or more days of any combination of walking, moderate-intensity, or vigorous-intensity activities, achieving a minimum total physical activity of at least 3,000 MET minutes/week.

Sample score days = 4 vigorous + 6 moderate + 4 walking = "at least 7 days." Total MET minutes/week = 2,315. As this is less than 3,000 the score does not qualify for high-intensity activity level.

Since this sample score has five or more days of any combination of walking, moderate-intensity, or vigorous-intensity activities, achieving a minimum total physical activity of at least 600 MET minutes/week, it qualifies as moderate-intensity level of activity.

Sample: Chapter 9
Brain Health Profile

Aim to increase the number of assets and reduce the number of risks across all categories

Category	Healthy	Borderline	Unhealthy	Asset	Risk	Maintain	Improve	Fix	Priority
Sleep	3	1U	1	3	2	2	1	2	2
Stress	1	2U	1	1	3	1	2	1	3
Social/ Mental	4	1U	1	4	2	3	2	1	1
Heart	4	1H	0	5	0	4	1	0	1
Physical	1	1U	1	1	2	1	1	1	1
Attitude	4	1H	0	5	0	4	1	0	1
Total	17	7	4	19	9	15	8	5	9

Note whether borderline activities are bordering on healthy (H) or unhealthy (U).

Sample: Chapter 9
Brain Health Plan

Category	Goal	Action	Steps	Target date (T) Achieved (A)
Sleep	1. Remove barriers to sleep 2. Get a regular sleep schedule	A technology-free bedroom	Find new place to charge my laptop and phone Don't bring devices into the bedroom ever Don't work from bed Buy an old-school alarm clock Set a bedtime alarm	T = 5/5/19 A = T = 6/30/19 A =
Stress	Get better life balance	Reduce time spent working by 15 percent	Do an audit on what I spend my time working on Factor outside breaks into my day Pursue my photography hobby	T = 9/30/19 A =
Mental/ social	Get more education	Take a night course	Research courses online. Save for fees—research grants. Register	T = 12/31/19 A =
Heart	Manage blood pressure	Consume a healthier diet	Reduce salt intake, get BP checked regularly	T = 5/15/19 A =
Physical	Sit less	Reduce sitting time by 20 percent	Set alarm on phone to remind me to get up and move. Do some routine activities standing	T = 7/1/19 A =
Attitude	Improve happiness levels	Smile more	Get my five-a-day	T = 5/30/19 A =

Notes

1   **Cognitive neuroscientist**—Cognitive neuroscience is a branch of both neuroscience and psychology that is concerned with the relationship between neural processes/systems in the brain and cognitive-behavioral processes and outcomes.

2   **Alzheimer's disease**—A neurodegenerative disorder characterized by the death of neurons in the hippocampus, cerebral cortex, and other brain regions. The earliest symptoms of the disease include: forgetfulness, disorientation to time or place, difficulty with concentration, calculation, language, and judgment. In the final stages, individuals are incapable of self-care and may be bedridden.

3   **Atrophy**—Wasting away of body tissue or organs, especially as a result of the degeneration of cells.

4   **Cognitive function (cognition)**—A group of mental processes that include attention, memory, producing and understanding language, learning, reasoning, problem-solving, and decision-making. **Cognitive decline** refers to a decline in the function or efficiency of cognitive function from one time point to another. **Mild cognitive impairment** refers to cognitive changes that are serious enough to be noticed but not severe enough to significantly interfere with day-to-day life. **Cognitive deficit** refers to impairment in an individual's mental processes that impact on how that individual acquires knowledge and understands and acts in the world. Clinically cognitively intact is when cognitive functioning is neither impaired nor deficient.

5   **Multiple sclerosis**—A progressive neurodegenerative disease that causes physical and mental disability as a result of damage to the central nervous system.

6   **Neuroplasticity**—Brain plasticity, or neuroplasticity, describes how experiences reorganize neural pathways in the brain. Long-lasting functional changes in the brain occur when we learn new things or memorize new information. These changes in neural connections are what we call neuroplasticity.

   Neuroplasticity occurs in the brain when:
   - the immature brain organizes itself at the beginning of life
   - the brain is injured, to maximize remaining function and compensate for lost function
   - in adulthood, any time something new is learned or memorized.

7   **Genetics**—Inherited characteristics.

8   **Brain volume**—A measure of brain size. The sum of the volumes of gray matter and white matter and often also cerebrospinal fluid.

9   **Neuronal networks**—A network of interconnected neurons (brain cells) in the nervous system.

10   **Cerebral cortex**—The thin layer of the brain that covers the outer part of the cerebrum, the most highly developed part of the brain. (Cerebrum comes from the Latin word meaning brain. It encompasses about two-thirds of the brain.) The cerebral cortex is divided into four lobes: frontal, parietal, occipital, and temporal.

11   **Molecule**—A group of two or more atoms bonded together that form the smallest fundamental unit of a chemical compound that can take part in a chemical reaction.

12 **Ventricles**—A communication network of cavities within the brain, filled with Cerebrospinal Fluid (CSF), which protects, bathes, and cushions the brain. The CSF that is made within this ventricular system helps to maintain chemical stability within the brain, removing waste products from cerebral metabolism and providing nutrients to nervous-system tissue.

13 **Locus coeruleus**—Located in the brain stem, the locus coeruleus is involved in the stress response and produces noradrenaline (norepinephrine), which plays a role in learning and memory. *Locus coeruleus* literally means "the blue spot," no prizes for guessing its color.

14 **Prefrontal cortex**—An area of the cerebral cortex that covers the front part of the frontal lobe.

15 **Cerebrospinal fluid (CSF)**—A liquid formed mainly in the ventricles in the brain that surrounds the brain and the spinal cord. CSF supports the brain, acts as a shock absorber, and provides lubrication between bones and the brain and spinal cord.

16 **Hypothalamus**—A complex brain structure that plays a vital role in many bodily functions and in maintaining optimal conditions.

17 **Autonomic nervous system**—The ANS, which has two components (sympathetic and parasympathetic), controls bodily functions including breathing, blood pressure, and heartbeat. A useful metaphor for the two components of the ANS is that one acts like an accelerator providing the body with a burst of energy to respond to the stressor (sympathetic) and the other acts like a brake calming, soothing, and pacifying the body after the threat has passed (parasympathetic).

18 **Adrenaline**—A hormone and a neurotransmitter that plays an important role in the fight or flight response.

19 **Thalamus**—A brain structure deep within the brain with multiple functions including relaying incoming sensory information to the appropriate areas of the brain for further processing.

20 **Parasympathetic nervous system**—Part of the autonomic nervous system. See 17 above.

21 **Classical conditioning**—A form of learning that involves associations between different events and stimuli. When a neutral stimulus (e.g., a bell) is paired with an unconditioned stimulus (e.g., food) which results in an involuntary response (e.g., salivating) the neutral stimulus (bell) begins to trigger a response (salivation) similar to that produced by the unconditioned stimulus (food).

22 **Noradrenaline**—A hormone and a neurotransmitter involved in mobilizing the brain and body for action.

23 **Dopamine**—A neurotransmitter involved in multiple functions including reward, pleasure, and movement.

24 **Sympathetic nervous system**—Part of the autonomic nervous system. See 17 above.

25 **Vitamins**—Complex organic compounds that are needed in small amounts by the body for normal growth and metabolism.

26 **Antioxidant**—A substance, such as vitamin E, vitamin C, or beta-carotene, thought to protect body cells from the damaging effects of oxidation.

27 **Oxidative stress**—Occurs when there is an imbalance between the production of free radicals and the ability of the body to counteract or detoxify their harmful effects through neutralization by antioxidants. Oxidative stress can lead to heart and blood vessel disorders, heart failure, heart attack, and neurodegenerative diseases including Parkinson's disease and Alzheimer's disease. Eating a balanced diet rich in vitamins, minerals, and antioxidants can protect the brain from oxidative stress.

28 **Cerebrovascular**—Relating to the brain and its blood vessels.

Bibliography

Chapter 1—Invest in Brain Health

Alzheimer's Disease International—Dementia Statistics. Retrieved from www.alz.co.uk/research/statistics.

Barnes, D. E., and Yaffe, K. (2011), "The projected effect of risk factor reduction on Alzheimer's disease prevalence," *Lancet Neurology* (9): 819–828. doi:10.1016/S1474-4422(11)70072-2.

Global action plan on the public health response to dementia 2015–2017. (2017), Geneva: World Health Organization. License: CC BY-NC-SA 3.0 IGO.

Gómez-Robles, A., Hopkins, W. D., Schapiro, S. J., and Sherwood, C. C. (2015), "Relaxed genetic control in human brains," *Proceedings of the National Academy of Sciences* 112 (48): 14799–14804. doi:10.1073/pnas.1512646112.

Mendis, S. (2013), "Stroke disability and rehabilitation of stroke: World Health Organization perspective." *International Journal of Stroke* 8 (1). https://doi.org/10.1111/j.1747-4949.2012.00969.x.

Norton, S., et al. (2014). "Potential for primary prevention of Alzheimer's disease: an analysis of population-based data," *Lancet Neurology*, Aug:13 (8). doi:10.1016/S1474-4422(14)70136-X.

Yusuf, S., et al. (2016), "Risk Factors For Ischaemic and Intracerebral Haemorrhagic Stroke in 22 Countries (the INTERSTROKE study): A Case-Control Study," *The Lancet*.

Chapter 2—Bank Reserves

Barnes, D.E., and Yaffe, K. (2011), "The projected effect of risk factor reduction on Alzheimer's disease prevalence," *Lancet Neurology* (9): 819–828. doi:10.1016/S1474-4422(11)70072-2.

Brookmeyer, R., et al., (2007),"Forecasting the global burden of Alzheimer's disease," *Alzheimer's & Dement.*, J. Alzheimer's Assoc. 3 (3): 186–191.

Chan, M. Y., et al., (2014), "Training older adults to use tablet computers: does it enhance cognitive function?" *The Gerontologist*. doi:10.1093/geront/gnu057.

Ferri, C. P., et al., (2006), "Global prevalence of dementia: a Delphi consensus study," *Lancet* 366 (9503): 2112–2117.

Ince P. G. (2001), "Pathological correlates of late-onset dementia in a multicenter community-based population in England and Wales," *Lancet* 357:169–175.

Katzman, R., et al. (1988), "Clinical, pathological and neurochemical changes in dementia: a subgroup with preserved mental status and numerous neocortical plaques," *Annals of Neurology* 23 (2).

Katzman R., et al. (1989), "Development of dementing illnesses in an 80-year-old volunteer cohort." *Ann Neurol.* 25: 317–324.

Kuiper, J. S., et al. (2015), "Social relationships and risk of dementia: a systematic review and meta-analysis of longitudinal cohort studies," *Ageing Research Reviews* 22: 39–57.

Landau, S., et al. (2012), "Association of lifetime cognitive engagement and low amyloid deposition," *Archives of Neurology*, 69 (5).

Middleton, L. E., and Yaffe, K. (2009), "Promising strategies for the prevention of dementia," *Arch. Neurol.* 66 (10): 1210–1215.

Miller, G. A. (1955), "The Magical Number Seven, Plus or Minus Two Some Limits on Our Capacity for Processing Information," *Psychological Review* 101, (2): 343–352.

Nyberg, L. M., et al. (2012), "Memory ageing and brain maintenance," *Trends in Cognitive Sciences* 16 (5).

Park, D. C., and Festini, S. B. (2017), "Theories of memory and ageing: a look at the past and a glimpse of the future," *J Gerontol B Psychol Sci Soc Sci*, 72 (1): 82–90. doi:10.1093/geronb/gbw066.

Pedditizi, E., Peters, R., and Beckett, N. (2016), "The risk of overweight/obesity in mid-life and late life for the development of dementia: a systematic review and meta-analysis of longitudinal studies," *Age and Ageing* 45 (1): 14–21. doi.org/10.1093/ageing/afv151.

Raz, N. (2000), "Aging of the brain and its impact on cognitive performance: integration of structural and functional findings," in F. I. Craik & T. A. Salthouse (Eds.), *The Handbook of Ageing and Cognition*, Mahwah NJ: Lawrence Erblaum Associates, 1–90.

Scarmeas, N., and Stern Y. "Cognitive reserve: implications for diagnosis and prevention of Alzheimer's disease," *Curr Neurol Neurosci Rep.* 4 (5): 374–380.

Stern, Y. (2002), "What is cognitive reserve? Theory and research application of reserve concept," *Journal of the International Neuropsychological Society* (8): 448–460.

Stern, Y. (2009), "Cognitive Reserve," *Neuropsychologia* 47 (10): 2015–2028. doi:10.1016/j.neuropsychologia.2009.03.004.

Stern, Y. (2012), "Cognitive reserve in ageing and Alzheimer's disease," *Lancet Neurol.* 11 (11): 1006–1012. doi: 10.1016/S1474-4422(12)70191-6.

Stern Y. (2017), "Cognitive ageing summit III." Retrieved from www.youtube.com/watch?v =V7e681vhr3w&index=4&list=PLmk21KJuZUM67-lwG7LY4LxGkgeblqMqY.

Strauss, E., Sherman, W. M. S., and Spreen, O. (2006), *A Compendium of Neuropsychological Tests Administration, Norms and Commentary*. Oxford University Press.

Tombaugh, T. N., Kozak, J., and Rees, L. (1999), "Normative Data Stratified by Age and Education for Two Measures of Verbal Fluency: FAS and Animal Naming," *Archives of Clinical Neuropsychology* 14 (2): 167–177.

von Bartheld, C. S., Bahney, J., and Herculano-Houzel, S. (2016), "The search for true numbers of neurons and glial cells in the human brain: A review of 150 years of cell counting," *J Comp Neurol.* 524 (18): 3865–3895. doi: 10.1002/cne.24040. Epub 2016 Jun 16.

Whalley, L. J., et al. (2004) "Cognitive reserve and the neurobiology of cognitive aging," *Ageing Research Reviews* 3: 369–382.

Wise, J. (2017), "Depression is not a risk factor for dementia, large cohort study concludes" *BMJ*, 2017; 357:j2409. doi: https://doi.org/10.1136/bmj.j2409.

Chapter 3—Cherish Sleep

Abel, T., et al. (2013), "Sleep, plasticity and memory from molecules to whole-brain networks," *Current Biology* 23 (17): R774–R788. http://doi.org/10.1016/j.cub.2013.07.025.

Eugene, A. R., and Masiak, J. (2015), "The neuroprotective aspects of sleep," *MedTube Science* 3 (1): 35–40.

Herculano-Houzel, S. (2013), "Sleep it out science," *Science* 18 (342): 316–317. DOI: 10.1126/science.1245798.

Krause, A. J., et al. (2017), "The sleep deprived human brain," *Nature Neuroscience Reviews* (18): 404–418.

Liu, Y., et al. (2014), "Prevalence of healthy sleep duration among adults" United States, MMWR Orb Mortal Wkly Rep 2016; 137–141. DOI: http://dx.doi.org/10.15585/mmwr6506a1.

National Sleep Foundation's Sleep Duration Recommendations. Retrieved 08/04/2018 https://sleepfoundation.org/press-release/national-sleep-foundation-recommends-new-sleep-times/page/0/1.

Pace-Schott, E. F., and Spencer, R. M. (2015), "Age-related changes in cognitive function of sleep" *Prog. Brain. Res* 191: 75–89; *Science* 3 (1): 35–40.

Paruthi, S., et al. (2016), "Recommended amount of sleep for pediatric populations: a consensus statement of the American Academy of Sleep Medicine," *J Clin Sleep Med* 12: 785–786.

Rasch, B., and Born, J. (2013), "About sleep's role in memory," *Physiological Reviews* 9 (2): 681–766. http://doi.org/10.1152/physrev.00032.2012.

Walker, M. (2017), *Why We Sleep: The New Science of Sleep and Dreams,* Penguin.

Witt, A. A., and Lowe, M. R. (2014), "Hedonic hunger and binge eating among women with eating disorders," *International Journal of Eating Disorders* 47 (3): 273–280. doi:10.1002/eat.22171.

Xie, L., et al. (2013), "Sleep drives metabolite clearance from the adult brain," *Science* 342 (6156): 373–377. doi: 10.1126/science.1241224.

Ybarra, O, et al. (2008). Mental Exercising Through Simple Socializing: Social Interaction Promotes General Cognitive Functioning. *Personality and Social Psychology Bulletin* 34 (2): 248–259. https://doi.org/10.1177/0146167207310454.

Chapter 4—Manage Stress

Arnsten, A. F. T. (2009), "Stress signalling pathways that impair prefrontal cortex structure and function," *Nature Reviews: Neuroscience* 10 (6): 410–422. http://doi.org/10.1038/nrn2648.

Chattarji, S., et al. (2015), "Neighborhood matters: divergent patterns of stress-induced plasticity across the brain," *Nature Neuroscience* 18: 1364–1375. doi:10.1038/nn.4115.

Garrido, P. (2011), "Ageing and stress: past hypotheses, present approaches and perspectives," *Ageing and Disease* 2 (1): 80–99.

Hueston, C. M., Cryan, J. F., and Nolan, Y. M. (2017), "Stress and adolescent hippocampal neurogenesis: diet and exercise as cognitive modulators," *Transl Psychiatry* 7 (4): e1081. doi: 10.1038/tp.2017.48.

Lupien, S. J., et al. (2009), "Effects of stress throughout the lifespan on the brain, behaviour and cognition," *Nat. Rev Neurosci.* 10 (6): 434–445. doi: 10.1038/nrn2639.

Marshall, P. J., Fox, N. A., and BEIP Core Group (2004), "A comparison of electroencephalogram between institutionalised and community children in Romania," *Journal of Cognitive Neuroscience* 16: 1327–1338. DOI:10.1162/0898929042304723.

Plassman, B. L., et al. (2011), "Incidence of dementia and cognitive impairment, not dementia in the United States," *Ann Neurol.* 70: 418–426.

Roozendaal, B., McEwen, B. S., and Chattarji, S. (2009), "Stress, memory and the amygdala," *Nature Reviews: Neuroscience* 10: 423–433. doi:10.1038/nrn2651.

Sandi, C., and Haller, J. (2015), "Stress and the social brain: behavioural effects and neurobiological mechanisms," *Nature Reviews: Neuroscience* 16: 290–304. doi:10.1038/nrn3918.

Sapolsky, R. M. (2015), "Stress and the brain: individual variability and the inverted-U.," *Nature: Neuroscience* 18: 1344–1346. doi:10.1038/nn.4109.

Schwabe, L. (2017), "Memory under stress: from single systems to network changes," *Eur J Neurosci.* 45 (4): 478–489. doi: 10.1111/ejn.13478.

Scott, S. B., et al., (2015), "The effects of stress on cognitive ageing," Physiology and Emotion (ESCAPE) Project, *BMC Psychiatry* 15: 1.

Chapter 5—Stay Social, Go Mental

"A Consensus on the Brain Training Industry from the Scientific Community" Max Planck Institute for Human Development and Stanford Center on Longevity, accessed 10/20/2018, http://longevity3.stanford.edu/blog/2014/10/15/the-consensus-on-the-brain-training-industry-from-the-scientific-community/.

Anderson, N. D., et al., (2014), "The benefits associated with volunteers among seniors: a critical review and recommendations for future research," *Psychological Bulletin* 6: 1505–1533. doi: 10.1037/a0037610.

Berkman, L. F. (1977), Social networks, host resistance, and mortality: A follow-up study of Alameda County residents. Doctoral dissertation. University of California, Berkeley.

Berkman, L. F., and Syme, S. L. (1979), "Social networks, host resistance, and mortality: a nine-year follow-up study of Alameda County residents," *American Journal of Epidemiology* 109: 186–204.

Brayne, C., et al. (2010), "Education, the brain and dementia: neuroprotection or compensation?," EClipSE Collaborative Members, *Brain* 133 (8): 2210–2216. https://doi.org/10.1093/brain/awq185.

Cacioppo, J. T., and Patrick, W. (2008), *Loneliness: Human Nature and the Need for Social Connection.* W. W. Norton and Company.

Cacioppo, S., Capitanio, J. P., and Cacioppo, J. T. (2014), "Toward a neurology of loneliness," *Psychological Bulletin* 140 (6): 1464–1504.

Cacioppo, J. R., Cacioppo, S., and Boomsma, D. I. (2014), *Cognition and Emotion*, 28 (1): 3–21. http://dx.doi.org/10.1080/02699931.2013.837379.

Davidson, R. J., and McEwen, B. S. (2013), "Social influences on neuroplasticity: stress and interventions to promote well-being," *Nature Neuroscience* 15 (5): 689–695.

Dunbar, R. (2009), "The social brain hypothesis and its implications for social evolution," *Annals of Human Biology* 36 (5): 562–572. doi: 10.1080/03014460902960289.

Fratiglioni, L., Paillard-Borg, S., and Winblad, B. (2004), "An active and socially integrated lifestyle in late life might protect against dementia" *Lancet Neurol.* 3 (6): 343–353.

Global Council on Brain Health (2017), "The brain and social connectedness: GCBH recommendations on social engagement and brain health," available at www.GlobalCouncilOnBrainHealth.org.

Hall, C. B., et al. (2009), "Cognitive activities delay onset of memory decline in persons who develop dementia," *Neurology* 73: 356–361.

Henry, J. D., et al. (2016), "Clinical assessment of social cognitive function in neurological disorders," *Nature Reviews Neurology* 12: 28–39.

Holt-Lunstad, J. et al. (2015), "Loneliness and social isolation as risk factor for mortality: a meta-analytic review," *Perspectives on Psychological Science* 10 (2): 227–237.

House, J. S., Robbins, C., and Metzner, H. L. (1982), "The association of social relationships and activities with mortality: prospective evidence from the Tecumseh," *American Journal of Epidemiology* 116: 1.

Kelly, M. E., Loughrey, D., Lawlor, B. A., Robertson, I. H., Walsh, C., and Brennan, S. (2014), "The impact of cognitive training and mental stimulation on cognitive and everyday functioning of healthy older adults: a systematice review and meta-analysis," *Ageing Research Reviews* 15: 28–43. doi: 10.1016/j.arr.2014.02.004.

Kelly, M. E., Duff, H., Kelly, S., Power, J. E., Brennan, S., Lalwor, B. A., Loughrey, D. (2017), "The impact of social activities, social networks, social support and social relationships on the cognitive functioning of healthy older adults: a systematic review," *Systematic Reviews* 6: 259.

Nucci, M., Mapelli, D., and Mondini, S. (2011), "Cognitive Reserve Index questionnaire (CRIq): a new instrument for measuring cognitive reserve," *Aging Clinical and Experimental Research* 24 (3): 218. DOI: 10.3275/7800.

Scarmeas, N., and Stern, Y. (2003), "Cognitive reserve and lifestyle," *J. Clin. Exp. Neuropsychol.* 25 (5): 625–633.

Shankar, A., Hamer, M., McMunn, A., and Steptoe, A. (2013), "Social isolation and loneliness: relationships with cognitive function during 4 years of follow-up in the English longitudinal study of ageing," *Psychosomatic Medicine* 75: 00Y00.

Stern, Y., et al. (1994), "Influence of education and occupation on the incidence of Alzheimer's disease," *JAMA* 271: 1004–1010.

Stern, Y. (2012), "Cognitive reserve in ageing and Alzheimer's disease," *Lancet Neurol.* 11 (11): 1006–1012.

Umberson, D., and Montez, J. K. (2010), "Social relationships and health: a flashpoint health policy," *J Health Soc Behav* 51 (Suppl): S54–S66. doi:10.1177/0022146510383501.

Chapter 6—Love Your Heart

Barnes, D.E., and Yaffe, K. (2011).

Cole, G. M., Ma, Q. L., and Frautschy, S. A. (2009), "Omega-3 fatty acids and dementia," *Prostaglandins, Leukotrienes, and Essential Fatty Acids* 81(0): 213–221. http://doi.org/10.1016/j.plefa.2009.05.015.

Gorelick, P. B., et al. (2017) "Defining optimal brain health in adults: a presidential advisory from the American Heart Association/American Stroke Association," *Stroke* 48: e284–e303. https://doi.org/10.1161/STR.0000000000000148.

Saver, J. L. (2006). "Time is brain—quantified," *Stroke* 37(1). DOI: 10.1161/01. STR.0000196957.55928.ab.

Topiwala, A., et al. (2017), "Moderate alcohol consumption as risk factor for adverse brain outcomes and cognitive decline: longitudinal cohort study," *BMJ* 2017; 357. doi: https://doi.org/10.1136/bmj.j2353.

World Health Organisation, Tobacco Free Initiative (TFI) fact sheet about health benefits of smoking cessation. Retrieved 7/25/18 from http://www.who.int/tobacco/quitting/benefits/en/.

WHO. A Global Brief on Hypertension (2013).

Chapter 7—Get Physical

Barnes, D. E., and Yaffe, K. (2011).

Buckley, J. P., et al., (2015), "The sedentary office: an expert statement on the growing case for change for better health and productivity," *Br J Sports Med*. (49): 1357–1362.

Driver, H. S., and Taylor, S. R. (2000), "Exercise and Sleep," *Sleep Medicine Reviews* 4 (4): 387–402. doi.org/10.1053/smrv.2000.0110.

Ebrahimi, K., et al. (2017), "Physical activity and beta-amyloid pathology in Alzheimer's disease: A sound mind in a sound body," *EXCLI J*. 16: 959–972. doi:10.17179/excli2017-475.

Ericksona, K. I., et al. (2011), "Exercise training increases size of hippocampus and improves memory," PNAS 108 (7): 3017–3022. www.pnas.org/cgi/doi/10.1073/pnas.1015950108.

Hamer M., and Chida, Y. (2009), "Physical activity and risk of neurodegenerative disease: a systematic review of prospective studies," *Psychol Med* 39: 3–11.

Hötting, K., and Röder, B. (2013), "Beneficial effects of physical exercise on neuroplasticity and cognition," *Neuroscience and Behavioral Reviews* 37: 2243–2257.

Kelly, M. E., Loughrey, D., Lawlor, B. A., Robertson, I. G., and Brennan S. (2014), "The impact of exercise on the cognitive functioning of healthy older adults: a systematic review and meta-analysis," *Ageing Research Reviews* 16: 12–31. DOI: 10.1016/j.arr.2014.05.002.

Levine, J. A., et al. (2005), "Interindividual variation in posture allocation: possible role in human obesity," *Science* 307 (5709): 584–586.

Office of Disease Prevention and Health Promotion (2015), www.healthypeople.gov/2020/topics-objectives/topic/physical-activity/national-snapshot?topicId=33.

Sofi, F., et al. (2011), "Physical activity and risk of cognitive decline: a meta-analysis of prospective studies," *J. Intern. Med*. 269 (1): 107–117.

Stamatakis, E., Hamer, M., Dunstan, D. W., et al. "Screen-based entertainment time, all-cause mortality, and cardiovascular events: population-based study with ongoing mortality and hospital events follow-up," *J Am Coll Cardiol* 57: 292–299.

Weuve, J., et al. (2004), "Physical activity, including walking and cognitive function in older women," *JAMA* 292 (12): 1454–1461. doi:10.1001/jama.292.12.1454.

International Physical Activity Questionnaire, Long Last 7 days, self-administered (2002), retrieved 4/21/2018. https://sites.google.com/site/theipaq/home.

Cuisle, F. "Exercise prescription for the prevention and treatment of disease. Scoring the International Physical Activity Questionnaire (IPAQ)."

Chapter 8—Adjust Your Attitude

Carstensen, L. L., et al. (2011), "Emotional experience improves with age: Evidence based on over 10 years of experience sampling," *Psychology and Ageing* 26: 21–33. doi:10.1037/a0021285. PMC 3217179.

Haslam, C., et al. (2012), "When the age is in, the wit is out: Age-related self-categorisation and deficit expectations reduce performance on clinical tests used in dementia assessment," *Psychology and Ageing* 27: 778–784. http://dx.doi.org/10.1037/a0027754.

Hecht, D. (2013), "The neural basis of optimism and pessimism," *Experimental Neurobiology* 22 (3): 173–199. http://doi.org/10.5607/en.2013.22.3.173.

Kemper, C. J., et al. (2011), "Measuring the construct of optimism-pessimism with single item indicators," paper presented at the 4th Conference of the European Survey Research Association (ESRA), Lausanne, Switzerland.

Levy, B. R., et al., (2002), "Longevity increased by positive self-perceptions of aging," *Journal of Personality and Social Psychology* 83: 261–270. doi: 10.1037/0022-3514.83.2.261.

Niedenthal, P. M., et al. (2010), "The simulation of smiles (SIMS) model: embodied simulation and the meaning of facial expression," *Behavioral and Brain Sciences* 33 (6): 417–433. doi: 10.1017/s0140525x10000865.

Robertson, D. A., King-Kallimanis, B. L., and Kenny, R. A. (2016), "Negative perceptions of ageing predict longitudinal decline in cognitive function," *Psychology and Ageing* 31 (1): 71–81. http://dx.doi.org/10.1037/pag0000061.

Radloff, L. S. (1977), "The CES-D scale: a self-report depression scale for research in the general population," *Applied Psychological Measurement* 1: 385–401.

Rossouw, P. (2013), "The neuroscience of smiling and laughter," *The Neuropsychothereapist* 1: 1.

Rylee, A. D. (2015), "Stereotypes of Aging: Their Effects on the Health of Older Adults," *Journal of Geriatrics*. http://dx.doi.org/10.1155/2015/954027.

Sebastiani, P., et al. (2013), "Meta-analysis of genetic variants associated with human exceptional longevity," *Ageing* 5 (9): 653–661.

Seligman, M. (2016), *Learned optimism: how to change your mind and your life*. Vintage Books.

Shimamura, A. P., Ross, J. G., Bennett, and H. D. (2006), "Memory for facial expressions: the power of a smile," *Psychon Bull Rev.* 13: 217–222.

Tsukiura, T., and Cabeza, R. (2008), "Orbitofrontal and hippocampal contributions to memory for face-name associations: the rewarding power of a smile," *Neuropsychologia* 46 (9): 2310–2319. doi: 10.1016/j.neuropsychologia.2008.03.013.

Warren, J. E., et al. (2006), "Positive emotions preferentially engage an auditory-motor 'mirror' system," *The Journal of Neuroscience* 26 (50): 13067–13075. doi: 10.1523/jneurosci.3907-06.2006.

Permissions

Grateful thanks to the authors and organizations that granted permission to reprint from the following:

Chapter 2
Figure 1
Reprinted from Stern, Y. (2012), "Cognitive reserve in ageing and Alzheimer's disease," *Lancet Neurol* 11 (11): 1006–1012. Copyright (2012), with permission from Elsevier.

Chapter 3
Figure 2
From Herculano-Houzel, S. (2013), "Sleep it out science," *Science* 18 (342): 316–317. DOI: 10.1126/science.1245798. Reprinted with permission from AAAS. Credit: V. ALTOUNIAN/SCIENCE.

Chapter 4
Assessment Perceived Stress (page 87): Perceived Stress Scale
Cohen, S., Kamarck, T., and Mermelstein, R. (1983), "A global measure of perceived stress," *Journal of Health and Social Behavior* 24: 386–396.

Used with the permission of the American Sociological Association, *Journal of Health and Social Behaviour* (1983) and Professor Sheldon Cohen, Carnegie Mellon University.

Chapter 5
Assessment: Social Connectedness (page 110): Berkman-Syme Social Network Index
Berkman L. F., (1977), Social networks, host resistance, and mortality: A follow-up study of Alameda County residents. Doctoral dissertation. University of California, Berkeley.

Permission to use the Berkman-Syme index granted by Professor Lisa Berkman, Harvard University.

Assessment: Loneliness (page 126)—UCLA Loneliness Scale
Hughes, M. E., Waite, L. J., Hawkley, L. C., and Cacciopo, J. T. (2004), "A Short Scale for Measuring Loneliness in Large Surveys: Results From Two Population-Based Studies," *Research on Aging* 26 (6): 655–672. Copyright © 2004 by (SAGE Publications).

Reprinted by Permission of SAGE Publications, Inc.

Chapter 8

Assessment: Happiness (page 209)

Reprinted by permission from Lyubomirsky, S., and Lepper, H. (1999), "A measure of subjective happiness: preliminary reliability and construct validation," Springer Nature: Social Indicators Research 46 (2): 137. Copyright © 1999, Kluwer Academic Publishers. Permission also granted by Professor Sonja Lyubomirsky, University of California Riverside.

Assessment: Life Orientation Test (page 212) — LOT-R

Copyright © 1994, American Psychological Association. Reproduced with permission. M. F., Carver, C. S., and Bridges, M. W. (1994), "Distinguishing optimism from neuroticism (and trait anxiety, self-mastery and self-esteem): a re-evaluation of the Life Orientation Test," *Journal of Personality and Social Psychology* 67: 1063–1078.

Permission granted by the American Psychological Association and Professor Michael F. Scheier, Carnegie Mellon University.

Assessment: Locus of Control (pages 214–15)

Rotter, J. B. (1966), "Generalised expectancies for internal versus external control of reinforcement," *Psychol Monogr* 80: 1–28.

Permission granted by Lindy Coldwell, University of Connecticut.

Assessment: Attitude to Aging Questionnaire — Short Form — (page 221)

Laidlaw, K., Kishita, N., Shenkin, S. D., and Power, M. J. (2018), "Development of a Short Form of the Attitudes to Ageing Questionnaire (AAQ)," *The International J. Ger. Psychiatr.* 33 (1): 113–121. Copyright © 2017 John Wiley and Sons Ltd.

Laidlaw, K., Kishita, N., Shenkin. S. D., and Power, M. J. (2017), "Development of a Short Form of the Attitudes to Ageing Questionnaire (AAQ)," *International Journal of Geriatric Psychiatry* 33 (1): 113–121. Reprinted by permission from John Wiley and Sons. Copyright © 2017 John Wiley and Sons Ltd and from Professor Ken Laidlaw, University of East Anglia.

Acknowledgments

This book was born of a brief encounter with a fellow guest, Graham Masterton, in the green room of an afternoon TV show. I'd been interviewed about brain health and sleep and he about his Katie Maguire novels. Graham not only introduced me to "the best literary agent in London" but he also became my mentor and friend. Graham, you are incredibly generous with your time, reading every word. This book, and I, have benefited immeasurably from your kindness, experience, wisdom, and wit.

Camilla Shestopal, you are indeed the best literary agent any writer could ask for. Thank you for having faith in me, for your critique and advice, and for working so hard on my behalf to find the perfect editor and publisher for this book. Amanda Harris, from our first meeting to final edits, your excellent, insightful, and practical suggestions have been invaluable. For a first time writer it has been fantastic to feel safe in your experienced hands. Grateful thanks to Ru Merritt for guiding me through the editorial process and to the rest of the talented team at Orion Spring and the Orion Publishing Group.

This book draws upon the work of many scientists whose endeavors over decades have increased our understanding of the brain and brain health. It has been an honor to share their work in these pages. I am sure that they would join me in acknowledging the thousands of research volunteers who give so freely of their time in the name of scientific advancement. Thanks also to those who fund my work and my supportive colleagues and collaborators, particularly those who worked on the Hello Brain, FreeDem, Brain Health For MS, and NEIL projects.

Thanks to Caoimhe for your eagle-eyed error spotting. Finally, special thanks to my husband, David, and sons Darren and Gavin and son-in-law Jamie for reading various drafts but mostly for your love, support, and inspiration. I may have ticked "write a book" off my bucket list, but be warned—the writing bug has bitten; there are more books to be written.